'If there is light in the soul,

there will be beauty in the person.

If there is beauty in the person,

there will be harmony in the house.

If there is harmony in the house,

there will be order in the nation.

If there is order in the nation,

there will be peace in the world.'

CHINESE PROVERB

Editorial Director: Jane O'Shea
Creative Director: Mary Evans
Project Editor: Lisa Pendreigh
Text Editor: Nicki Marshall
Picture Researcher: Nadine Bazar
Production Controller: Tracy Hart

First published in 2002 by
Quadrille Publishing Ltd
Alhambra House
27–31 Charing Cross Road
London WC2H 0LS

Cataloguing-in-Publication Data: a catalogue record
for this book is available from the British Library.

ISBN 1 903845 83 1

Printed in Hong Kong.

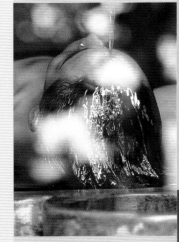

insight 6

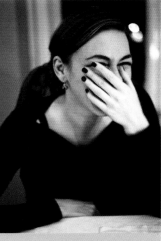

laughter 10

enhance 32

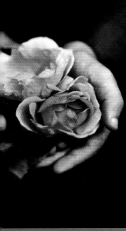

enrapture 62

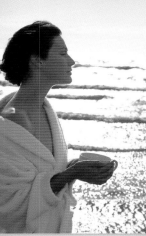

stillness 82

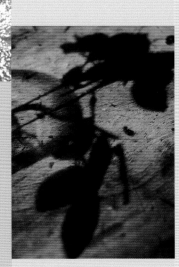

balance 102

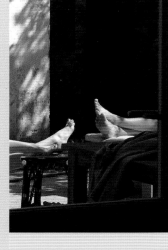

escape 132

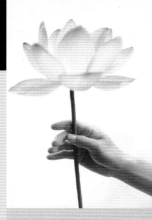

inspire 148

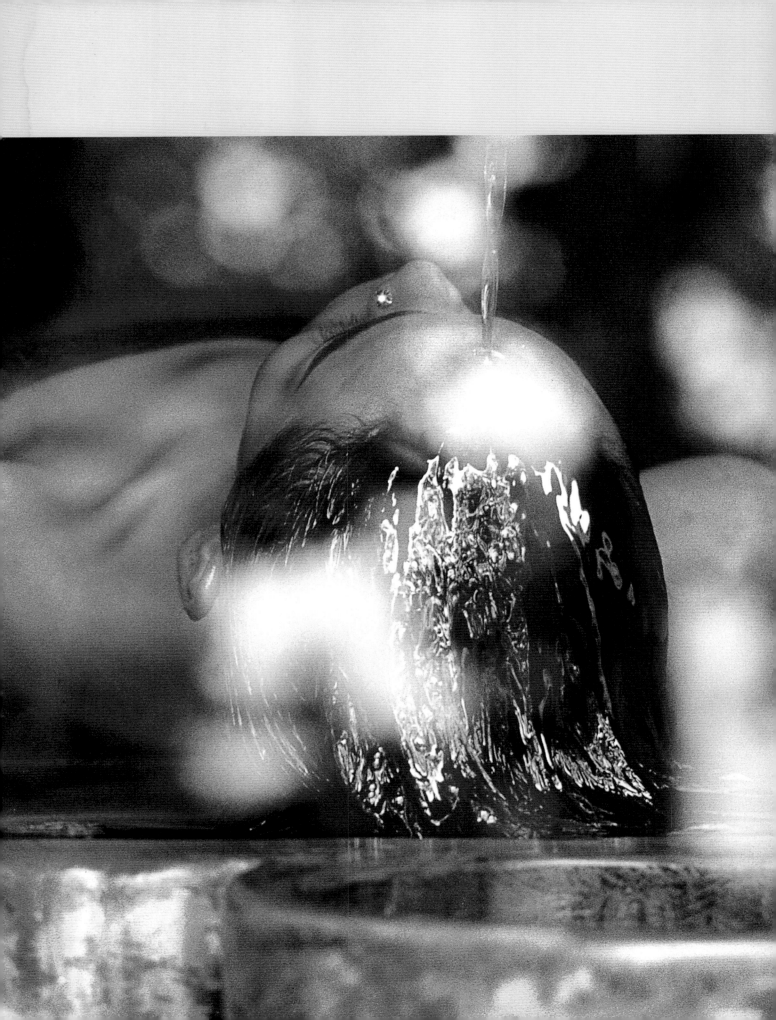

insight

In the frenetic, stressful, work-oriented society in which we live it is easy to lose sight
of what is important and disregard our own place in the world. To be truly happy, to
enjoy all that life has to offer, we need to rediscover our sense of self-worth,
acknowledge who we are and what is important to us, and strive to become who we
want to be. Creating a balance between work and the rest of life can require some
financial sacrifice; however length and quality of life, peace of mind and lightness of
spirit, and freedom from pain and disability belong to a completely different realm of
values. By treating ourselves well, through diet, stress control, exercise and nurturing,
we can create our own opportunities to live well and enjoy every waking moment:
bringing laughter and joy into all that we do; enhancing our beauty and appreciating
our individuality; being enraptured by sensual pampering; creating stillness and
calm in our minds; finding balance and harmony within; escaping and finding peace
in ourselves.

We all have the potential to improve spiritually, physically and mentally, but we must work to develop the tools and skills to do so. This takes discipline, daily practice and self-love: feeding ourselves foods that make us feel well; inhaling aromas that have positive emotional and psychological benefits; creating living and working spaces that are pleasing to the eye and comforting to the spirit; tending our bodies with a loving touch; dressing ourselves in clothes that both look and feel good; exercising to work the body and invigorate the mind; giving ourselves space and time to relax and escape; spending more time in nature; adopting a positive outlook and looking for the beauty and good in everything rather than focusing on the problems.

Sensory awareness plays a huge role in how we conduct our lives and the pleasures we derive from it. Colour and light can be revitalising, calming or nurturing and we can make use of these different properties to enhance specific areas of our lives. We can create sensory stimulation in our homes by using materials and substances with varying textures and temperatures and can feel comforted and reassured by therapeutic touch. We can use fragrance to enhance or change our mood, lift our spirits and calm our nerves. Food flavours can boost our energy levels or induce relaxation. We can lift our spirits or re-energise by listening to music and bring peace to our hearts with silence.

The greatest beautifiers in the world are health and happiness. Regardless of age, a smile, a twinkle in our eye and a spring in our step will announce to the world that we are young at heart and great fun to be with. Laughter creates joy in our lives, evoking beneficial physical and chemical changes in the body that promote wellbeing. Every religion teaches us that the face and the body are reflections of what is inside: unpleasant thoughts can make even the most naturally beautiful person ugly, whereas positive energies bring unparalleled radiance. Inner beauty can only shine through when we are at peace with ourselves. Along with this doctrine comes the ability to accept that improving ourselves is the only way to achieve long-lasting happiness. For this we have to make the most of ourselves by highlighting our assets – physical, spiritual and emotional – and working on our flaws.

Changing ourselves for the better can only benefit our relationships with others and may lead to those around us changing too. We are individually responsible for our lives. We have choices. Much of the stress we suffer comes from the fear that we will make mistakes, choose a wrong path or upset others. We need a strategy for life. We should be mindful of every action so that each is undertaken with full understanding and responsibility for its consequences. We need to find personal courage to help us overcome adversity without compromising ideals and generosity towards others. Pursuing our dream should never be at the cost of anyone else.

If we have an implicit belief in our ability to make things better then we will achieve our goal. Exercise brings our body and mind together and, as we get fitter, improves our self-esteem so that we have greater faith in our own abilities. Prayer and meditation concentrate our life force on something outside ourselves and invite positive thoughts. When we are still, when we calm our breath, we become conscious of our inner selves. Contemplating the beauty of nature, the landscape, the flowers, and the seasons that are so magical, reminds us that there is power all around us and that our problems are insignificant.

Achieving happiness is a holistic process that requires change in every part of our lives. To begin on this road we need to recognise where we are now and locate our desired destination. Only then can we start taking small steps to get there. Each one of us has a personal route that we can create and fine tune as we progress on the amazing, sensory journey of life. We should take time to explore everything around us and enjoy the sights, sounds, tastes, scents and textures that stimulate our senses and enrich our experiences. It is never too late to find your way – let your journey begin today.

laughter

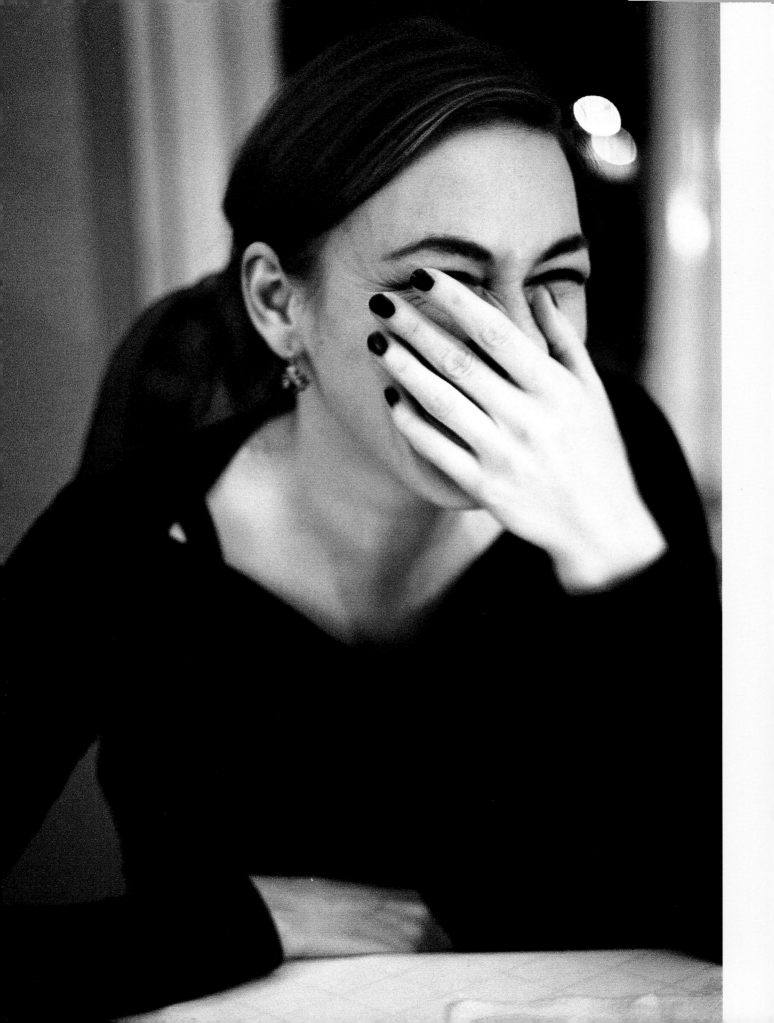

laughter

Each morning when we awake we tune into our senses and prepare to meet the world in search of fulfilment. The first thought of every day should be positive; before rolling out of bed, try to think of something good, something that makes you smile. Spend some time at the start of the day before the onslaught begins, focusing on each part of you. Put goals into perspective, relax the body, make the spirit receptive and open the mind – only then can we perform at our best.

The importance of a healthy lifestyle, with daily exposure to fresh air and sunlight and good nutritional habits cannot be overemphasised. This sounds easy but how many of us really do it? How much better do you feel after an early morning run, a brisk thirty minute walk in the park, or after a stimulating ashtanga yoga session which warms up the joints, leaving you with increased energy levels and a warm, satiated glow.

The world around us is rich with colour that is too often overlooked. Colour and natural light have significant impact on us – in the very early morning before sunrise green rays prepare and harmonise the energies for the day ahead. At sun up yellow stimulates us to rise in the morning, fresh and well rested and helps us work with a clear and uncluttered mind.

Sound can have a curiously uplifting effect on the emotions. Playing upbeat happy music from Cesaria Evora never fails to bring a smile to my lips. The Cuban piano maestro Ruben Gonzalez adds a spring to my step and of course we must never discount the raw energy of the flamenco guitar from the Gypsy Kings to get things moving.

Fresh, vibrant scents awaken the senses and recharge us for the day ahead. Shower gels infused with the zingy tang of lemon, lime or grapefruit make the early morning bathing routine a sensory delight. For an added energy boost create a perfumed oil to massage onto your skin after showering or dab onto pulse points for an instant lift; try fresh citrus notes of bergamot and lime essential oils in a neutral oil base.

Breakfast provides us with essential body fuel but should also exercise the taste buds; take time to enjoy the flavours and textures of the first meal of the day. Taste the tang of your favourite fresh fruit in a smoothie or combine the clean, yet tart, taste of natural yoghurt, with the sweet vitality of seasonal berries.

It is easy to be enthusiastic and energetic if you have something to look forward to – so try to plan a fun element into every day. Celebrate your family and friends and take pleasure in spending time with them. Rediscover the joys of going out to 'play' like you did as a child and go to the movies, the park, the ice rink, an open-air concert. To enjoy life is all that we can ask for – so throw back your head and laugh.

scents for stimulation

Essential oils can have a profound influence on the psyche. Energising, refreshing oils such as rosemary, peppermint and the citrus oils – bergamot, lemon, lime and grapefruit – offer an instant boost. They encourage good circulation, aid detoxification and help to increase concentration and clarify thoughts.

There is much that we can do to enhance our daily performance and wellbeing through the vaporisation of essential oils. The Japanese have become masters of aromacology in the workplace, which they use to increase productivity and create a happier working environment: rosemary is the office hero, boosting concentration and memory, whilst increasing energy and stimulating brain activity. Lemon comes a close second for its mind-sharpening abilities and help with learning. As the afternoon draws on, or when tensions are high and tiredness is kicking in, clary sage and marjoram can assist in clear thinking. Simply add up to 4 drops of essential oil to a water-filled diffuser or oil burner and allow the fragrant vapours to fill the air.

The tiny molecules of essential oils enter the body both by absorption through the skin into the bloodstream and by inhalation into the lungs. Oils can be added directly to water in an oil burner for inhalation, but for application to the body they should always (with the exception of lavender) be diluted in a vegetable-based carrier oil or neutral cream.

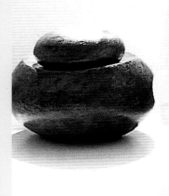

We can also choose our deodorants and perfumes more carefully to get the full benefit of natural fragrances. Deodorants often contain aluminium salts, alcohol and chemicals that block pores; seek out those that use refreshing essential oils such as antiseptic tea tree and eucalyptus and astringent rosemary. Complimentary therapists often recommend crystal deodorants because they do not impede the lymph system around the breast area.

Personal fragrances make an impact on how your day starts and different scents can influence your mood. How you feel about yourself will also influence your choice of scent: green, floral fragrances appeal to women with an assertive air – think of freshly cut grass and ivy leaves; woody scents are best suited to lively, spirited women with a zest for life and a love of the great outdoors. A fragrance may not have the same effect on you throughout the four seasons, particularly heavy scents which can be too heady and dramatic for summer, so choose two or three distinct scents that can work their magic at different times of the year.

Once you are bathed and fragranced it's time to get dressed. With your sense of wellbeing enhanced, and your body energised, you should feel ready to take on the day.

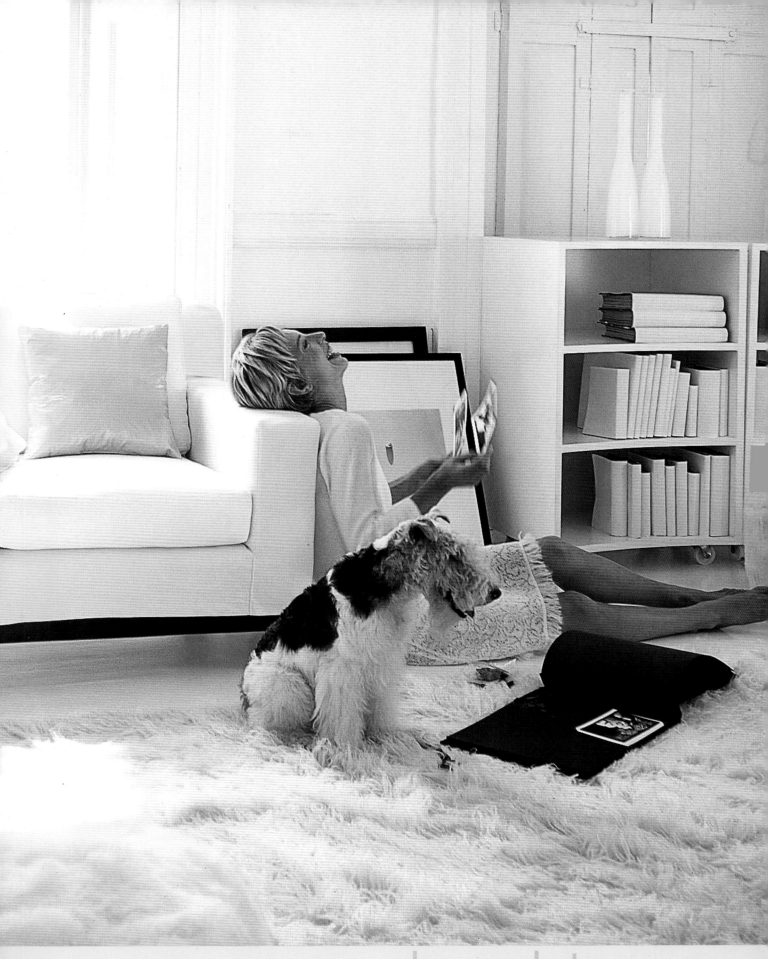

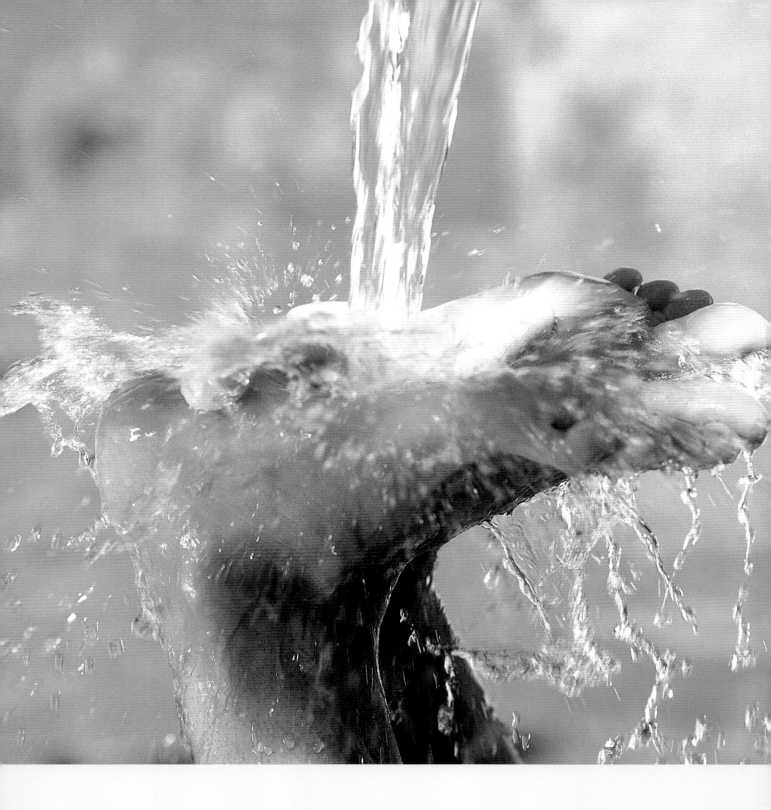

laughter

early-morning energy boosters

From the first moment of waking everything that you do affects your health, state of mind and energy levels. Use the time before breakfast to set yourself up for the day ahead; try to find a routine that you really enjoy so that it lifts your spirits while increasing your energy.

Early-morning revitalisation of the body and soul takes many forms. Exercise is a great way to start the day but can require an abundance of self-discipline, at least at the start, until the released endorphins kick in or the visible results become too good to ignore. Luckily there are also some quick-fix skin re-energisers that take minimal preparation time, have real benefits and are a pleasure to wake up to.

dry body brushing

This is the perfect method for attaining super-smooth, glowing skin that tingles all over and feels full of life. Brushing stimulates the body's nervous system and the circulation of the blood and lymph whilst exfoliating the skin, which makes it particularly good for anyone suffering from poor circulation, dry skin, 'goose-flesh' skin and fatigue. Use it as the prelude to your early-morning bathing routine.

EQUIPMENT REQUIRED

A dry body brush

Using a gentle, wrist-flicking motion softly brush your skin all over with short strokes, starting from your shoulders and working downward. Always brush towards the heart and start each limb at the closest point to the trunk so that the lymph portals open and the lymph can flow freely. For example, when brushing an arm start at the shoulder and work your way down – always flicking the brush toward the shoulder – until you reach the fingertips. Then each light stroke should be long, running all the way up the arm to the shoulder. Make sure the brushing is light enough not to redden the skin or you may simply disperse the lymph that lies just underneath.

Any extra preening and pampering you can do during your bathing routine entirely depends on how much time you have each morning. I like to make time for all my favourite treatments as often as I can – all too soon I'm caught up in the business of the day but I feel much more focused and ready to face the world when my mind and body are full of vitality.

For a very simple early-morning wake-up we can all learn from the Scandinavians. This stimulating reviver works well in either a bath or shower, but if you prefer to bathe or don't have access to a shower take an empty jug into the bathroom with you. Step into a warm bath or shower and massage the body well, until you feel gently relaxed. If you are in a shower turn the water to cold and stay underneath it for as long as you can bear. For those in a bath, fill up your jug with cold water and pour this over you, as many times as you can. This final cold rinse really makes the brain realise it's awake and kick-starts the body for the day's activities.

early-morning energy boosters

revitalising body scrub Body scrubs are one of my perennial addictions; they are truly stimulating and my skin always feels refreshingly rejuvenated. This early-morning skin re-energiser will set you up for the week ahead. It sloughs away the surface layer of dead cells that dull the skin's surface and leaves your skin supercharged and radiant. Indulgent and aromatic. This shower scrub can soon become addictive, although you shouldn't use it more than twice weekly. Neither should it be used if you are pregnant, or immediately before sun exposure or after shaving.

TO PREPARE AND USE THE SCRUB

Place a generous handful of Dead Sea salts in a bowl and add the following customised oil blend:

30ml sweet almond oil
4 drops grapefruit essential oil
4 drops lime essential oil
2 drops rosemary essential oil

Due to the different densities of the ingredients, the mixture will separate when left to stand; before use, swirl the scrub with your fingertips to ensure the oils are well integrated with the Dead Sea salts.

Use your hand to massage the scrub in circular movements over wet skin, from the soles of the feet working upward all over the body. Pay particular attention to rough, dry areas such as knees and elbows.

The oils can make the shower or bath slippery under foot so take care.

When the salt grains start dissolving in the scrub it is time to thoroughly rinse under warm water. Step out of the shower or bath carefully and envelop yourself in a warm, fluffy towel. Relax for a few minutes before patting your skin dry.

This scrub is highly moisturising so there is no need for further body creams or lotions.

laughter

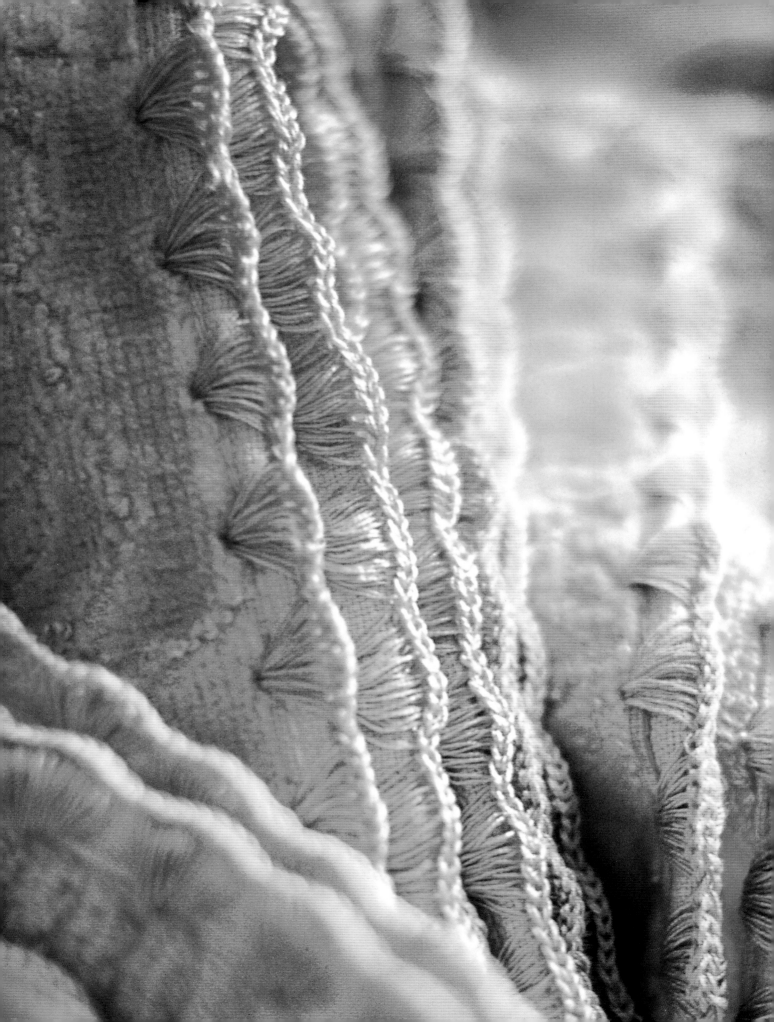

When time is limited in the mornings a high-pressure hot shower does wonders for the body. For a particularly refreshing and exfoliating shower, use a body wash infused with a citrus essential oil and scrub all over with a specially textured Japanese washcloth, which has been designed for easy back scrubbing. As a general rule, choose shower gels with skin moisturising, smoothing and tightening properties such as regenerative herbal oat extract, hydrolysed wheat protein, skin-softening aloe vera and seaweed extracts; try to avoid the harsh surfactant sodium lauryl sulfate, which is, unfortunately, a common ingredient in many soaps and washes.

energising self-massage

After your morning bath, a self-massage is a wonderful way to start the day. Massage improves the circulation, encourages the lymphatic drainage system and the elimination of toxins from the body. It also raises energy levels, moisturises the skin and heightens our own bodily awareness and sense of touch. Take your time to work all over your body so that every part of you feels alive. Try customising your regular massage oil or body cream with essential oils to enhance the sensory experience.

TO PREPARE AND USE THE MASSAGE BLEND

30ml carrier oil (such as jojoba or evening primrose) or a neutral nourishing body cream
10 drops (in total) bergamot, lavender, juniper and/or peppermint essential oils

Warm a little of the massage oil blend or body cream between the palms of your hands each time you apply it to a new area of the body.

Always massage in the direction of your heart to help the blood and lymph to flow.

Beginning with your feet, massage them with your thumb using circular motions and working from your heels down to your toes.

Next work up your legs from the heels, to the calves, to the thighs, to the buttocks. Use the heel of your hand to work in circular movements over any areas of tension.

Placing your hands on either side of your spine at the base of your back, stroke firmly upward as far as you can reach.

Now concentrate on your abdomen; with the palm of your hand gently circle the belly using a clockwise motion.

From there, gently and rhythmically squeeze your arms, starting at the wrists and going upward. Then, using the palm of your hand, massage with firm circular movements from the wrists to the shoulders.

Now grasp the flesh on either side of your neck and firmly knead, working from the neck to the shoulders.

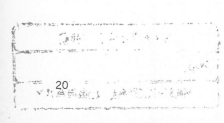

Starting from the base of the skull, place your fingers on each side of your neck and again firmly knead down as far as possible until you reach your shoulders.

To complete your massage, place the flat of your left hand anywhere on your right foot and the flat of your right hand anywhere on your left foot.

This creates a calming positive–negative charge on the body, which helps release stiff muscles and wakes up the nervous system. After a count of twenty, slowly withdraw your hands.

Take a few minutes to relax and enjoy the feeling of energy circulating through your body.

early-evening re-charger Sometimes we have evening commitments we feel too lethargic to face. Whenever you feel like this don't just give in and curl up on the sofa; take a little time to recharge your batteries and you'll soon be raring to go. When time is available this bath is a great way to get rid of some of the surface tension and give the soul a booster charge for the evening ahead.

TO PREPARE AND USE THE BATH SOAK

Stir 2 tablespoons Epsom salts or Dead Sea salts into a hot bath to gently ease away fatigue, aches and pains. This can be especially welcome after a hard day at work or after vigorous exercise.

To maximise the spiritual effects of the bath and for sensual stimulation, add the following customised oil blend to the water:

30ml almond oil
3 drops each basil, juniper and grapefruit essential oils

Before getting into the tub, swirl the water to ensure the oils have been thoroughly distributed.

Lie back and soak for up to 20 minutes. Close your eyes and breathe deeply to inhale the invigorating fragrant vapours, transporting them to the mood centre of the brain.

laughter

21

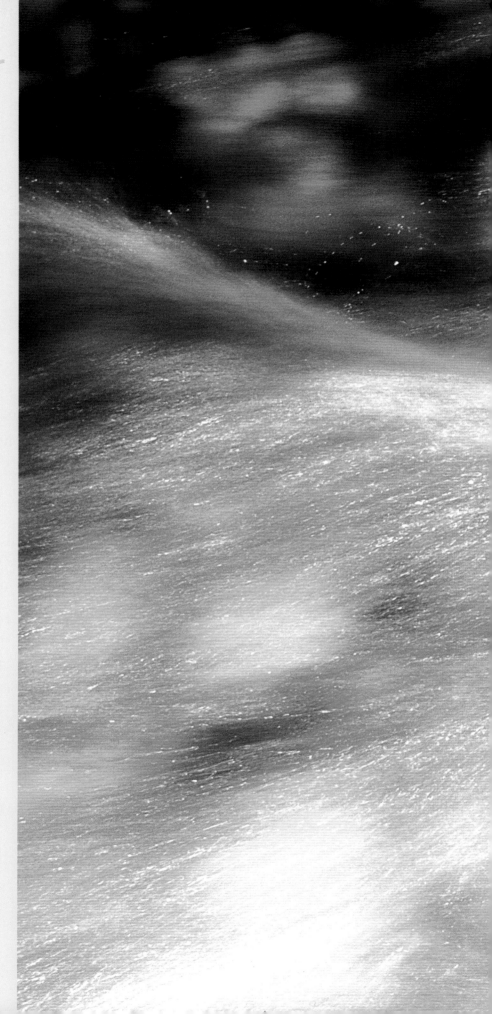

laughter

'What you are is what you
have been.
What you will be, is what
you do now.'

BUDDHA

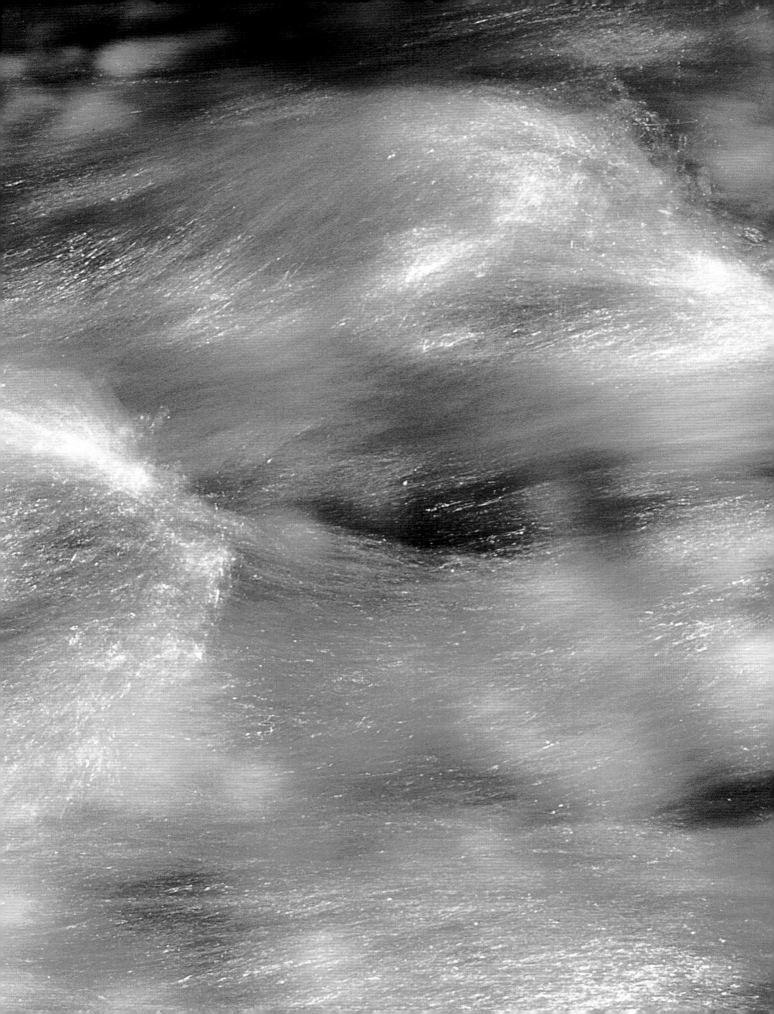

exercise for energy

Energy generates energy: there is no beauty routine more rewarding than an exercise programme which firms the body, increases resistance to disease, develops our ability to handle stress and makes us feel vibrant and youthful. The fitter you are the more active you will be. For a wonderful way to start your day try exercising outside in the morning sun; go for a jog, a bike ride or a brisk walk through the park, or just go down into the garden and do a few rounds of sun salutations. Take this opportunity to reconnect with the sights and sounds of the world around you.

Exercise regularly: your body was built to move, so use it or lose it. Exercise slows heart disease by improving vascular reactivity; it is like taking heavy-duty anti-oxidants. It helps lower the amount of adrenaline circulating in the body, reducing the effects of stress. The physical release relaxes the whole body and it also gives the mind a rest and promotes good sleep. Lean body mass is increased through exercise, greater muscle mass increases metabolism and improves the ratio of good to bad cholesterol in the blood.

Choose a form of exercise you enjoy doing so you will be motivated to keep going. Concentrate on what you do like about working out – whether it be the 'exercise glow', the feeling of virtue, the freedom of movement, the increased energy, the improved spirits, the pleasant tiredness afterward, the deep sleep – and that thought will keep you going. Just remember, well-toned muscles, and the lower percentage of body fat that comes with them, make us look young, healthy and strong; vanity can be the best motivator of all.

Choose recreation over a nose-to-the-grindstone gym workout whenever possible – do the original activity rather than the gym imitation. Reconnect with that playful spirit from childhood; have fun with your friends. Establish the exercise habit: set realistic goals; seek out activities that make you feel good and with which you are comfortable; be honest with yourself; keep yourself entertained; if possible recruit a workout partner whose level of fitness is similar to your own; keep track of your training; set goals and reward yourself generously. Just get outside and do something and build from there. There are 3 basic areas of exercise that are necessary for maintaining general fitness.

cardiovascular This is the most important of the three areas as it determines the ability of the heart, lungs, blood, blood vessels and tissues to deliver and use oxygen. It also creates muscular strength and endurance, flexibility, balance and agility. The effort you put into a cardiovascular programme determines your body composition or ratio of fat to lean tissue, which changes over time and is dependent on your lifestyle. Just 20 minutes of cardiovascular exercise three times a week is all that is required for basic aerobic fitness. Forty minutes four to six times a week can take your fitness to the next level. Vary your activity to stave off boredom: if you can no longer face jogging then hop on to a bicycle, hit the cardio machines in the gym, swim in the pool, walk in the park or go dancing.

weight training The older we get the more our lifestyle determines our wellbeing. Strength training is the most effective form of exercise in reversing the quintessential marker of age, frailty. People lose 30 per cent of their strength between the ages of 50 and 70, with a further 30 per cent every decade thereafter – a frightening thought. Regular weight-bearing exercise is now considered a more important factor than calcium intake in preventing and arresting osteoporosis. By developing muscular strength and endurance you have increased control over your movement, so that you move your body safely and efficiently. Ideally weight

laughter

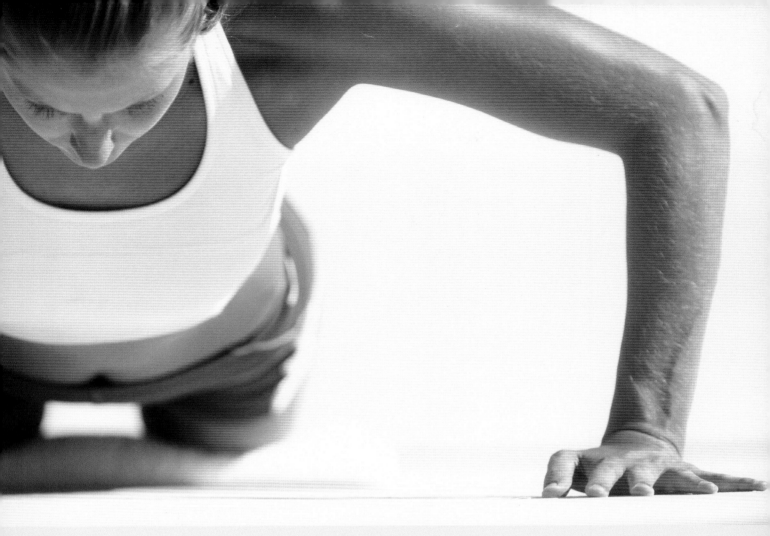

training should be undertaken at least twice a week, working the core four muscle groups with three sets of 8 to 12 repetitions per exercise, increasing the weight if 12 repetitions do not take you to muscle failure.

The chest and front of shoulders (anterior deltoids) and the back of the upper arms (triceps) – the most popular exercise to work these is the bench or chest press.

The upper back (latissimus dorsi) and the back of the shoulder (posterior deltoid) – work these areas with pull downs or single arm rows.

The buttocks (gluteus maximus), thighs (quadriceps) and backs of thighs (hamstrings) – work these areas simultaneously with squats and lunges.

The abdominals – crunches are the most beneficial exercises for the stomach muscles.

Weight training is not the only way to get strong. There are many other extremely effective techniques. Callisthenics, Pilates and yoga, in which the body

works against gravity, also have substantial benefits. Resistance bands are great for travel when you do not have easy access to a gym.

Callisthenics are now back in vogue; these are part of the old-fashioned, boot-camp way of exercising that you may remember from PE lessons at school – push ups, pull ups, squats and crunches.

flexibility A flexible body is a comfortable body; we feel better emotionally when our muscles are relaxed and our joints bend freely. Flexibility is vital for stress reduction. Stretching reduces tension in the muscles and should be done before, and immediately after, all exercise sessions.

To be agile your heart and lungs should be efficient, your muscles strong, your whole body supple and your balance fine-tuned. As we lose our agility we grow less adaptable, more awkward and prone to accident and we begin to feel less pleasure in our physicality.

eat for energy

Eating is one of life's great pleasures and it is sad that in our culture of abundance so many people have developed unhealthy relationships with food. It does not have to be this way; eating well will enhance your physical health and increase your total enjoyment of life. Eating should be a pleasurable experience, so enjoy it – savour the aromas wafting from the kitchen, delight in the different tastes of each part of the meal and feel the distinct textures as you munch blissfully away.

Awareness is one of the best innate tools we have to control appetite and instil a sense of enjoyment in eating. We need to remind ourselves why we eat and become aware again of when and what we are eating; **we need to experience textures and tastes and get in touch with appetite and hunger**. Before every meal clear and quieten your mind; breathe deeply once or twice and focus your thoughts on your food. Eat slowly, as this allows you to become more aware of the sensory pleasure of food. It will also give your brain the chance to recognise the fact that your hunger is being satisfied, which means there is less chance of overeating.

Genetics, health and medical history, eating preferences and lifestyle all influence our nutritional needs. Assess your personal needs or goals. Consider the balance of your meals and ensure you have a variety of foods, including generous amounts of vegetables and fruit, moderate amounts of protein-rich foods and whole grains, and small amounts of healthy fats and oils. **Food is fuel: the quality of the food we put in our bodies affects the way they run.** Choose fresh seasonal vegetables and fruit, food free from additives, preservatives, hormones and other unnecessary chemicals. Buy organic whenever possible and discover great tastes coupled with the rewards of supporting a cleaner and safer environment. A balanced approach to eating energises the body, stimulates the mind and enriches the spirit.

Eat regularly throughout the day to prevent extremes in hunger that lead to fatigue and over-eating; eat every three to five hours and work towards a pattern of breakfast, lunch and dinner and an afternoon snack if necessary. Know yourself, learn how to maximise your energy and minimise your hunger. Learn to distinguish physical hunger from hunger associated with stress, anxiety or sadness. **Vaporising essential oils can often satisfy a false appetite,** imparting a sense of nurturing. Oils with natural appetite-suppressing qualities include tangerine, lemongrass, rose, jasmine, peppermint, vanilla and orange.

Different foods are digested and absorbed at different rates and raise blood sugar levels accordingly. Simple sugars (found in processed and refined foods) cause blood sugar to rise in a way that demands a surge of insulin, giving us a quick rush but no lasting energy.

They can also cause body tissue to become puffy and capillaries near the surface of the skin to expand, creating redness and blotchiness. On a grander scale over-consumption of these sugars can lead to diabetes, raised blood pressure and elevated levels of bad cholesterol. Eating less carbohydrate-rich food helps maintain lower blood sugar levels; however restricting them too much may leave you without enough fuel. Emphasise wholegrains which provide fibre, vitamins and minerals and help keep blood sugar levels stable for hours after consumption. Other good sources of carbohydrates include beans, sweet potatoes, barley and wholegrain pasta cooked al dente.

Limit the amount of sugar in your diet and avoid sweeteners. Be sensible about salt as it constricts and tightens tissue and dries out both the skin and hair; if consumed in excess it inhibits energy flow and hardens fat and cholesterol deposits in the body. Instead, **pamper your palate with delectable herbs and spices** like calming rosemary, warming cinnamon and invigorating ginger (also anti-inflammatory and a digestive aid).

Try to include protein-rich foods, such as beans, soy foods and fish, in every meal as they help to control hunger and stabilise energy levels. Beware of consuming too much animal-derived protein as it decomposes rapidly in the body producing a build-up of toxins (such as ammonia and uric acids), which can place tremendous stress on the kidneys and the intestines. An excess of animal protein can also deplete calcium and mineral reserves and promote the accumulation of protein on the surface of the body in the form of warts, moles and calluses.

Certain oils and fats are critical for healthy hair, skin and nails, and for keeping the body running smoothly, but it is recommended that they should only amount to 20–30 per cent of our daily calories. The type of fat is as important as the amount: emphasise monounsaturated fats found in extra virgin olive oil, canola oil, avocados, olives and nuts. Have a daily source of omega-3 fat in your diet, this is found in flaxseeds, walnuts and pumpkin seeds as well as cold-water fish such as salmon, trout, mackerel and herrings. Saturated fats and cholesterol can unnaturally age the skin, making it inflexible and prone to wrinkles, so choose low-fat or fat-free milk, yoghurt and cheese, skinless poultry and the leanest, most trimmed cuts of red meat. Avoid hydrogenated fats such as margarine; instead use oils that are liquid at room temperature.

Most importantly of all, drink plenty of water – at least eight glasses every day. The human body is about 70 per cent water and it is crucial that we replenish the supply. **Think water first,** and then supplement your daily fluid intake with fruit juice mixed with water and refreshing herbal tea or, even better, green tea. Black tea is also rich in antioxidants but all caffeinated beverages trigger fluid loss, as does alcohol, so drink at least an extra half cup of water to compensate for each cup of these culprits.

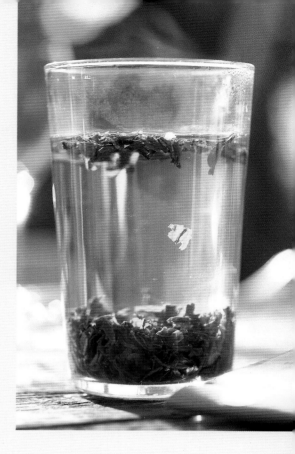

stimulating herbal tea For those who rely on strong coffee to get through the day, there are natural alternatives that can give you a gentle wake up without the injection of caffeine into the system. This tea can also help to increase mental alertness on a day when you are feeling sluggish.

TO PREPARE THE TEA

1 ½ cups water
½ teaspoon crushed fennel seeds
1 teaspoon dried rosemary leaves
honey (to taste)

Bring the water to the boil, add the fennel seeds, reduce the heat and simmer for 10 minutes.

Pour the fennel infusion over the rosemary leaves, cover and steep for 5 minutes.

Strain and sweeten with honey to taste.

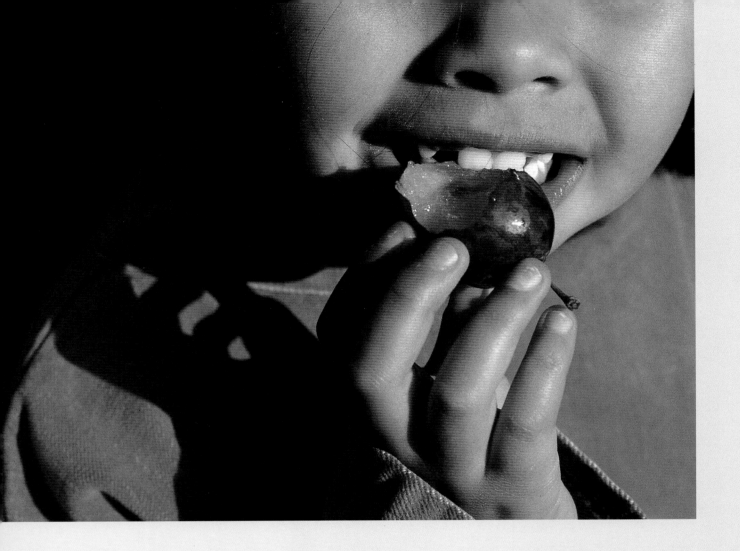

energy foods
Including raw foods in our diet increases energy and helps us digest and eliminate all our other food. Vegetables and fruit are the best source of many of the properties we need to sustain energy levels and maintain general health: they fight cancer and diabetes, protect the heart, boost the immune system and are antioxidants; they also have phytochemicals (the biologically active substances that protects plants from too much sunlight, blight and pollution), which enhance and protect human health. Vitamins and minerals in fruit and vegetables are often bound on to other nutrients that help absorption. For example, bioflavonoids, which are found in the pith of citrus fruit, aid the absorption of vitamin C. Eating eight to ten servings of vegetables and fruit each day will give your body vital fuel. A serving is one piece of fruit or half a cupful of an item.

laughter

BRIGHTLY COLOURED FRUIT AND VEGETABLES offer extra health benefits: red, yellow and orange vegetables and fruit are rich in antioxidants such as carotenoids, lycopene and lutein that neutralise free radicals and prevent regenerative diseases such as cancer and heart disease; dark green, leafy vegetables are rich in antioxidants and in fibre for intestinal health; dark red, blue and purple fruit and vegetables are rich in antioxidants such as phenols and in terpenes that help boost the immune system and have anti-carcinogenic properties.

ALLIUMS – such as onions, garlic, leeks and shallots – are rich in organosulful compounds, which produce enzymes that detoxify potential carcinogens. They are also rich in phenols, which have antiviral and anti-inflammatory properties. Garlic can reduce the stickiness of blood platelets, helping to prevent the kind of clot that can lead to heart attacks, and may also reduce the risk of hardening of the arteries.

CRUCIFEROUS VEGETABLES – such as cabbage, kale, cauliflower, brussels sprouts and broccoli – are rich in indoles and isothiocyanates that block cancer-causing agents from reaching cells.

LEGUMES are rich in fibre for intestinal health and in protease inhibitors, flavonoids, and saponins, which help prevent heart disease and cancer and enhance the immune system.

CITRUS FRUITS are rich in limonene, which helps prevent cancer and heart disease; carotenoids, such as beta carotene, lycopene, and lutein; the flavonoid hesperedin, particularly noted for fighting breast cancer; and perillyl alcohol, which helps boost the immune system.

GRAPES are loaded with ellagic acid, which blocks the body's production of enzymes that cancer cells need to grow. They also contain antioxidant phenols that may prevent blood clots. Red grape skins also contain resveratrol, a natural fungicide that slows the build up of bad cholesterol.

FLAXSEED is rich in fibre that promotes intestinal health, and in lignans, a phytoestrogen that helps promote beneficial intestinal bacteria and may help alleviate mild menopausal symptoms.

SOY BEANS AND SOY PRODUCTS are rich in the phytoestrogens genistein and daidzein, and in the protease inhibitor BBI, which provides protection against cancer.

laughter

vital vitamins

Juicing is a quick way to benefit from raw fruit and vegetables and enhance beauty, health and general wellbeing. Juices provide a wealth of vitamins, minerals and other nutrients, which cleanse and balance the body. The juices of all fruit and vegetables hold stores of pure water that has already been filtered through their complex structures making them easier on our digestive systems.

Juices on their own will not bring perfect health but their contribution cannot be over-estimated: all fruits contain acid that can help remove toxins from the digestive tract; green vegetables are rich in cleansing chlorophyll, which is why watercress and spinach can be so helpful on a detox programme; and carrot and tomato can act as a tonic to the liver. Always try to use mature, ripe, organic produce and drink your fresh juice just after making it, or at least during the same day, to ensure maximum nutrient content. Add fresh herbs (coriander, mint, oregano, marjoram and basil), ground spices (ginger, nutmeg, cinnamon), honey for a little sweetness, wheat germ for a boost of B-complex vitamins, plain live yoghurt to assist the digestive system or semi-skimmed milk to turn your juices into shakes. For an extra energy boost of potassium add a mashed banana or avocado to the blend.

Start by drinking up to three 250ml glasses of juice a day, but over time you can increase this to six glasses. Drink vegetable and fruit juices to get the maximum nutritional benefit – too many of the latter will overload your system with fructose causing a rapid rise in blood sugar – but avoid mixing vegetable and fruit juices together in the same glass, the only exceptions being carrot and apple which both go well with most other vegetables and fruits.

Make sure that you dilute dark green vegetable juices (broccoli, spinach and watercress) and dark red vegetable juices (beetroot and red cabbage) by four parts juice to one part filtered or mineral water.

Try the following combinations to get you started, but do not forget to keep eating whole fruit and vegetables too. Each combination makes approximately one large glass of juice. Dilute with water if you prefer.

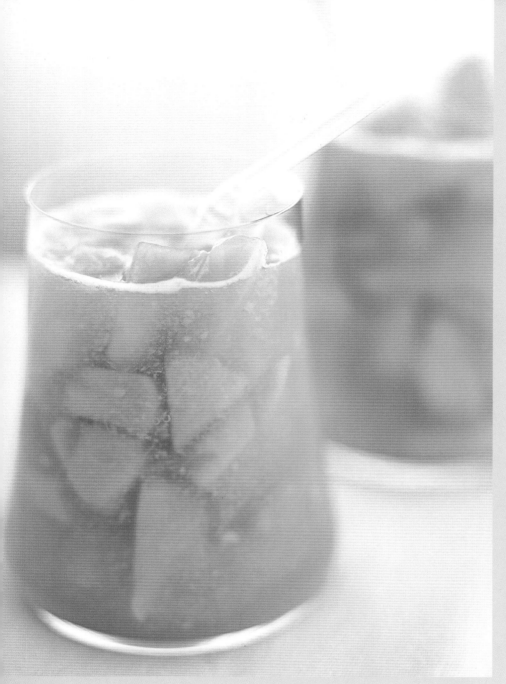

all-round goodness

2 large carrots
1 mango or 1 medium cantaloupe melon
or
2 large carrots
8 small broccoli florets
1 chunk cucumber

alert and active

1 ½ large carrots
7 large spinach leaves
2 stalks celery

beauty boost

½ lettuce
3 stalks celery
2 tomatoes
or
2 large carrots
15 large spinach leaves
1 avocado, mashed

energy enhancer

1 mango
½ pineapple
1 banana mashed
¼ pint milk or small pot plain yoghurt
1 teaspoon desiccated coconut
½ teaspoon honey

enhance

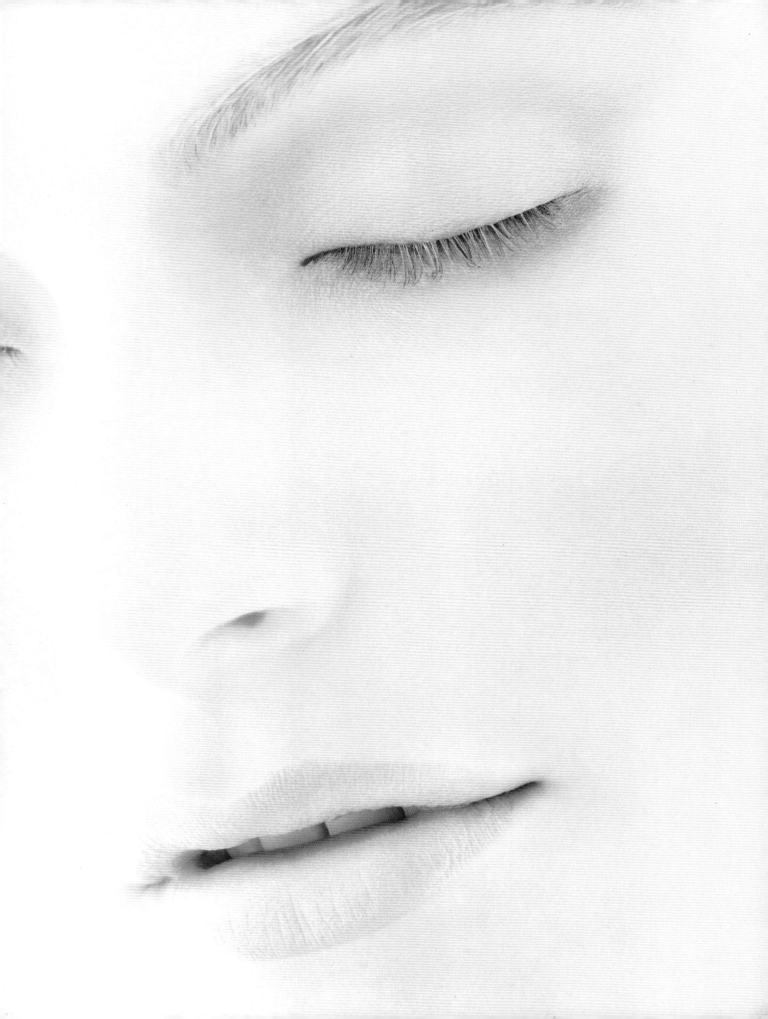

enhance

The universal concept of beauty at any age is youthful, clear radiant skin, sparkling eyes, healthy shiny hair and a positive attitude to life. Make-up, the right clothes and personal grooming combine to provide the finishing gloss. Beauty exists in every one of us but it needs to be discovered and highlighted. We all have potential to enhance our beauty, beginning with a daily practice of self-awakening, self-realisation and self-appreciation. Be true to yourself rather than slavishly following magazines and pandering to the aesthetic ideals of your peers – discover your own signature sense of style and celebrate the real you.

Many women spend very little daily time caring for themselves, believing it to be a selfish thing. However, a skincare regime should be regarded as a necessity not a luxury. We need to take care of ourselves and need to believe that we are worth the attention. We will only find beauty in ourselves by accepting who we are and cherishing all those little things that make us unique. A healthy attitude to food, exercise and body image will bring a healthy glow to our cheeks and uncover our real beauty.

Our daily activities, our emotions and the food we consume all have an effect on our health. Living a healthy life should not be a chore, it should be an inspiration. Along with our daily 1.5 litres of water we should also enjoy plenty of fresh fruit and vegetables to keep our skin, eyes, hair and nails healthy. Ripe, organic, seasonal produce offers all the essential vitamins and minerals while stimulating our senses with their fresh, vibrant aromas, rainbow colours and exciting array of textures and flavours.

As beauty and health mirror our lifestyle we need to ensure that the environments in which we live and work are as pleasant as possible: if either makes us feel uncomfortable, unhappy or even unwell, it will affect our general wellbeing. Take time to try and create a happy and positive environment to enhance your health and your life. In your home, use textures, materials and colours that comfort you and allow you to relax and be yourself; at work, personalise your space by adding elements that inspire you, nurture you or boost your confidence. Use the delicate aromas of essential oils and the deep resonance of music and sound to promote a sense of peace within yourself, which will encourage you to believe that your body and soul are worth looking after.

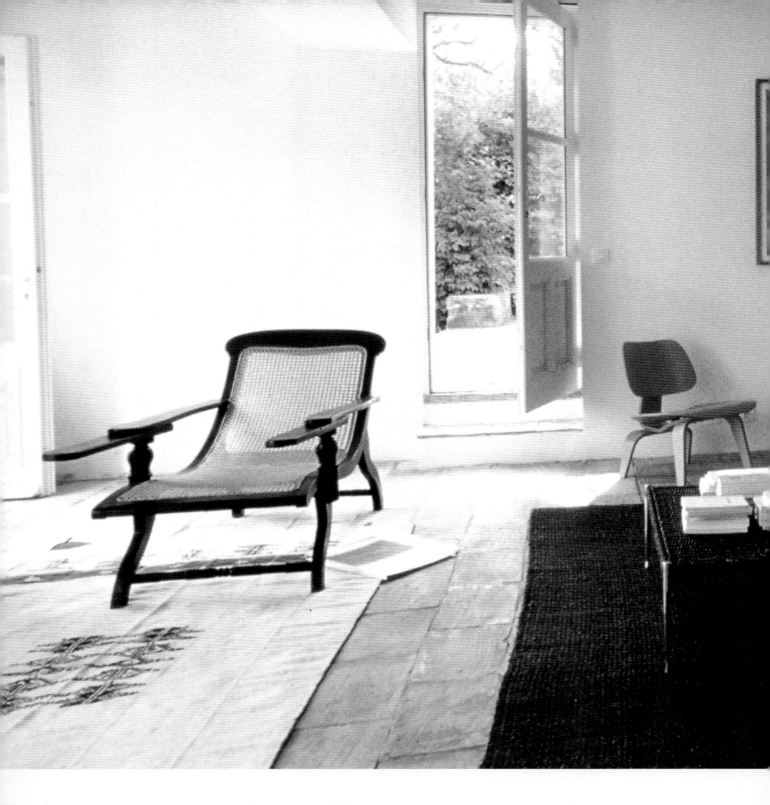

home harmony
The environments in which we spend our lives are as important to our general health as looking after our physical and emotional needs. A happy, nurturing home and an energising, positive workplace will lift our spirits and calm our minds.

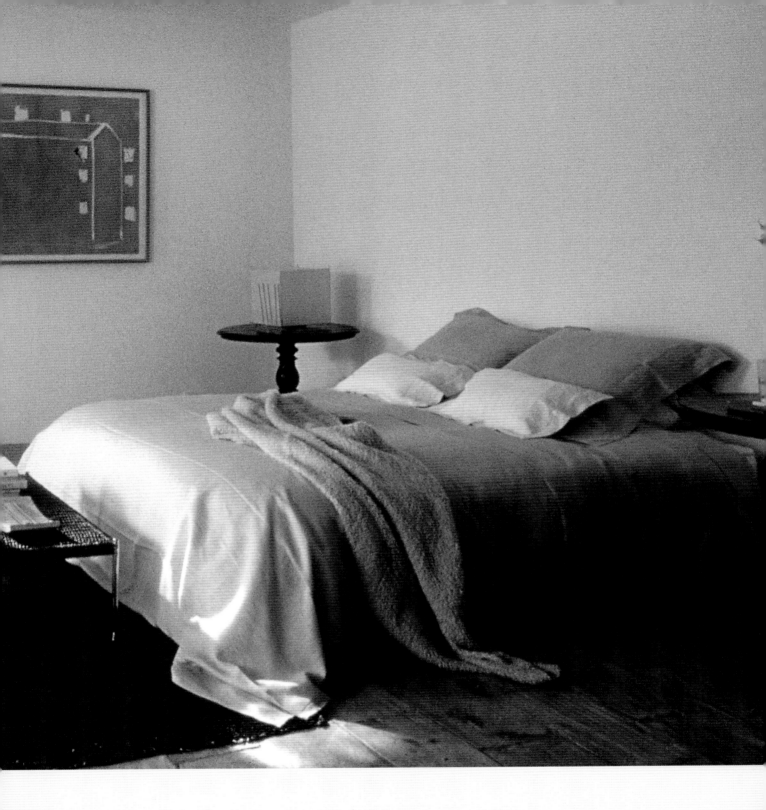

enhance

daily delights

Make a few subtle changes in your daily routine to increase your sense of wellbeing and enhance your life. Even the most subtle, simplest of things can make a real difference and help to ease you through the day.

Minimise stress during journeys to and from work by introducing aromatherapy, even if it consists of a few drops of essential oil on a tissue that you can inhale periodically: lavender is wonderfully balancing as it energises without being too stimulating; rosemary is good for concentration should tiredness kick in during a long drive home; geranium promotes peacefulness and calms anxiety.

At lunchtime take a mental break away from your work; after a respite we are often more productive. Settle down, ideally away from your desk, to eat a nutritious, well-balanced lunch and savour every mouthful. Allocate part of your lunch break to some movement. Going for a walk revitalises your mind and body, assists digestion and allows you to reflect upon your achievements of the day and evaluate your remaining tasks.

Keep a soothing rosewater spray on your desk so you can periodically refresh your face with this delightfully cooling and relaxing aroma. Mid-afternoon, when the drop in blood sugar hits, try burning energising essential oils, such as lime, rosemary or lavender, or a combination of olibanum and frankincense to enhance creativity. Do some breathing exercises. Take a short walk to clear your mind and reawaken your body.

Winding down is an essential part of a balanced day. Before leaving work list all tasks that you need to achieve tomorrow so that you can leave with a clear mind. Upon arrival home in the evening shed the clothes, and the concerns, of the working day. Burn tangerine or rose essential oils to create a calm, nurturing atmosphere. Perhaps now is the time for some light yoga, a walk in the park, a bike ride or a leisurely, de-stressing, aromatic soak in the tub.

Dinnertime should be for sharing food and conversation; acknowledge and cherish these special moments. Softly play some heart-warming background music like Ella Fitzgerald, Billie Holiday or Dean Martin. Light candles, lay the table with your favourite pieces, dim the lights, savour each carefully prepared mouthful and enjoy the company of your nearest and dearest. Finish the meal with relaxing chamomile or peppermint tea to aid digestion. Enjoy every comforting moment.

Before bedtime retreat to your own special place to meditate and take a few minutes to reflect on the day. Take a leaf out of Far Eastern cultures and fragrance your bedroom prior to sleep: spray a dilution of your favourite essential oil onto your bed linen; add a sachet of lavender inside your pillow case; gently diffuse 4 drops of relaxing lavender essential oil or sandalwood in a water-filled oil burner and practise some deep abdominal breathing before dropping off. Consciously work to end the day with genuine peace of mind.

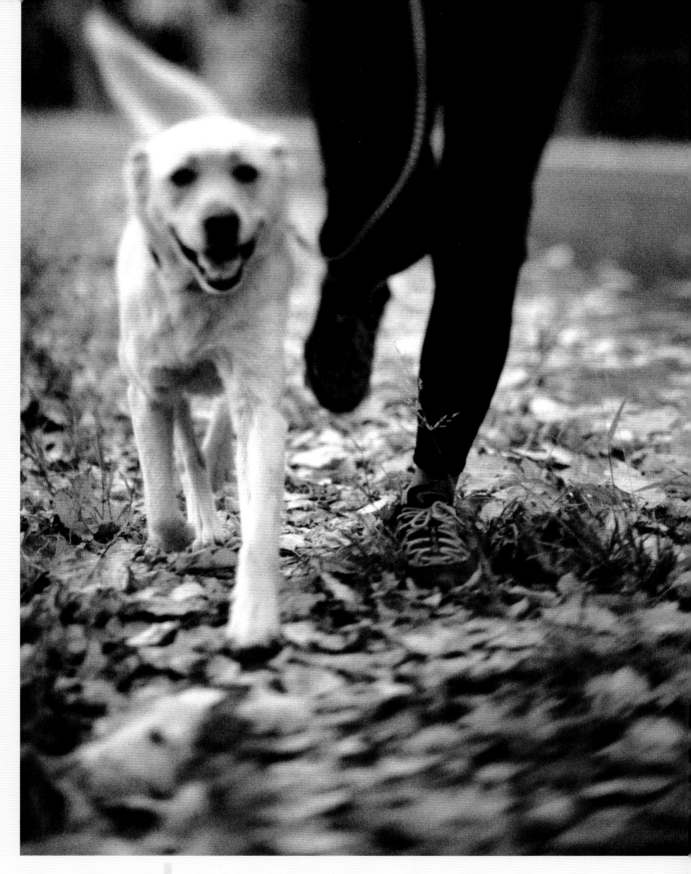

enhance

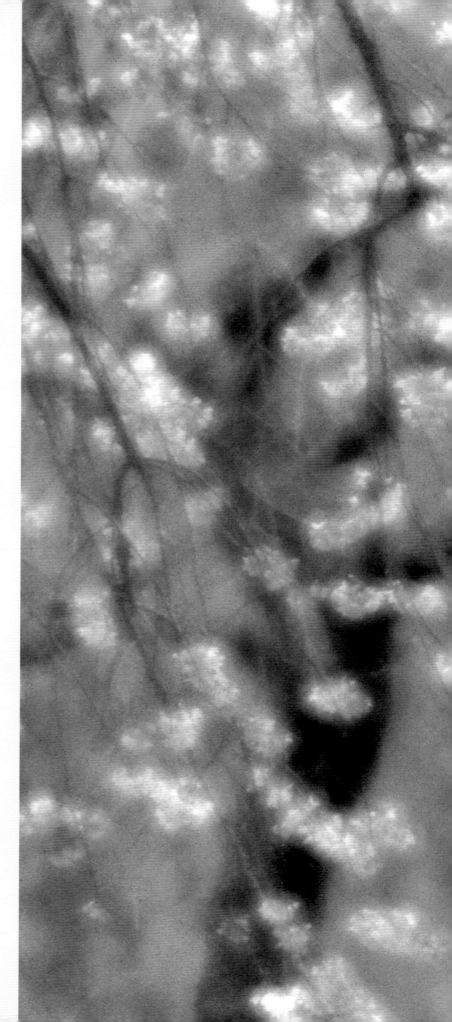

enhance

'To love oneself is

the beginning of a

life-long romance.'

OSCAR WILDE

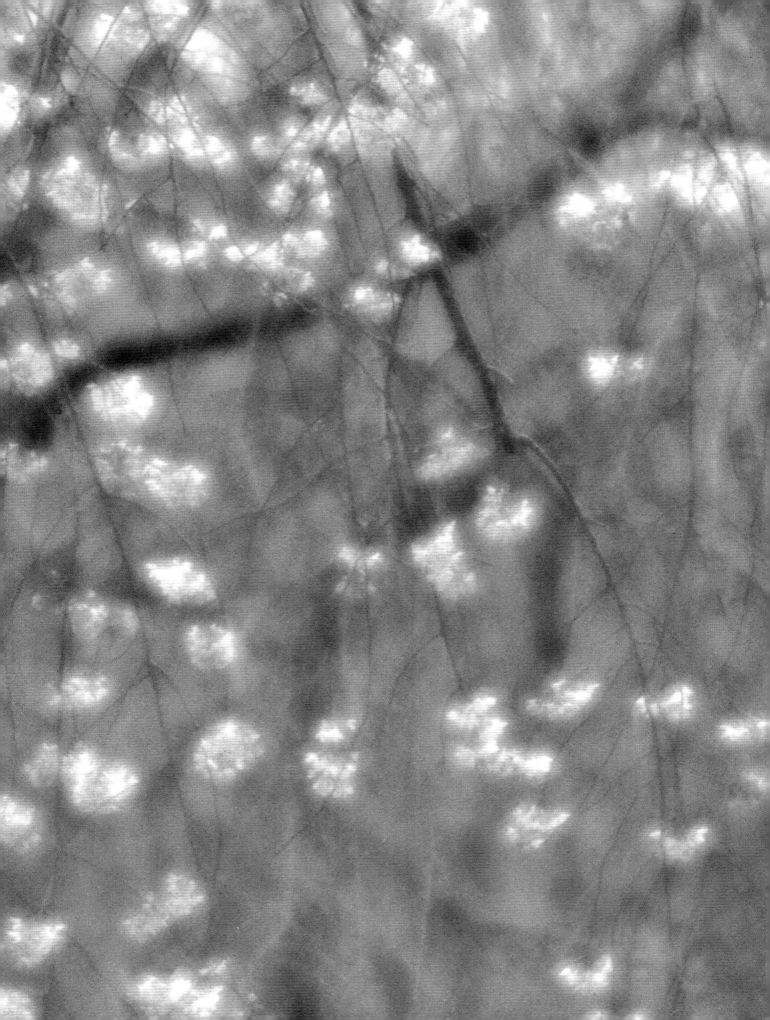

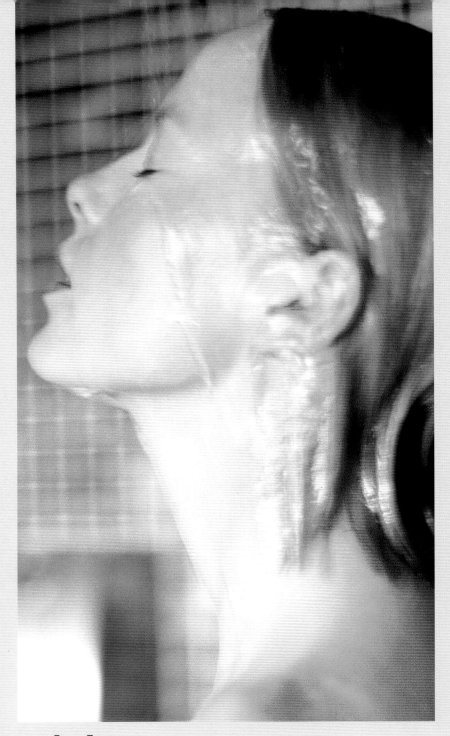

essential skincare

One of the pre-requisites of beauty is healthy, smooth skin with a flawless complexion. This should not be regarded as a sign of vanity but as a mark of self-respect. How much better do we feel about ourselves if our skin is clear and soft and our eyes are bright? Getting into the habit of a good skincare routine early in your life means that your skin will already be well prepared for the day when fine lines start appearing. Skin is one of our most precious assets. Be kind to your skin and it will repay you tenfold in return by maintaining its smoothness, colour and vitality much longer.

With the onslaught of pollution, stress, bad eating habits and overwork it is all important that we develop routines to keep the face and body looking radiant and youthful for as long as possible. Two of the most important requirements for skin are fresh air and plenty of water – our bodies are 70 per cent water and of that 35 per cent is found in the skin. There can be little dispute that drinking at least 1.5 litres a day of pure water at room temperature has a positive effect on the skin. If your skin is behaving badly it can be a sign that your whole system is overloaded with stress or toxins.

In younger women skin renews itself every 2–3 weeks, but as we age this process takes up to twice as long. Skin ageing occurs when the major components of its underlying support structure, collagen and elastin, degenerate. This is mainly due to damage by ultra violet light and free radicals, both of which cause the collagen fibres to twist and mat so the skin begins to line, wrinkle and sag. Most sun damage has already taken place by the time we are 18 so early rigorous sunscreen use cannot be over-emphasised. From the age of 50 the number of elastin fibres decline, oil production diminishes, the skin can no longer hold water and the rate of cell renewal is reduced. The sooner we start taking care of our skin the better we can face the inevitable progression of nature. Oestrogen is an important skin regulator and promotes supple, soft, healthy skin. As oestrogen levels decline dramatically at menopause, hormone-replacement therapy is noted for putting the glow back into skin. This is now an area that many skincare houses are investigating to see how similar effects can be synthesised using plant-derived compounds.

Skin uses 7 per cent of the oxygen we inhale; it also absorbs a small amount directly through its pores. It is important, therefore, to let the skin breathe by spending a part of each day bare. The best time to do this is overnight: apply your night cream, allow it to sink in for twenty minutes and then blot any excess off with a tissue before going to sleep – the cream will have done most of its work then the skin can breathe until morning.

Exercising in the open air in the least polluted place you can find is the best way of oxygenating the skin. During exercise oxygen surges to every cell in your body, allowing more efficient absorption of nutrients and faster cell growth. This means higher collagen production, which in turn leads to improved skin texture and moisture

retention and a thicker, more resilient epidermis. Research has shown that the more oxygen you take in the less likely you are to suffer from free-radical damage.

Exercise also stimulates circulation, prompts a sluggish digestive system to eliminate toxins and waste (pasty, blotchy, blemish-ridden skin being the tell-tale signs) and brings a radiant glow to the complexion. A daily walk in fresh air, however cold the weather, improves circulation and gives the skin a healthy glow. The sun offers vibrational nutrients, vitamins A and D and helps our brain to produce serotonin, which is the key to feeling happy. Protection is needed against strong sun or wind as regular exposure to either accelerates the signs of ageing. Sun-damaged skin is dry on the surface and displays increased pigmentation marks over time, coupled with a premature loss in firmness and increased wrinkles. In oily skin it may manifest itself in excess sebum production and spots. Dermatologists are now recommending we wear daily sun protection of at least SPF15 even in cities during winter. Look out for creams that also contain antioxidants, which protect the skin against damage from pollution.

A clean skin is a vehicle for moisture exchange; if this function is hampered and the toxins produced by the body are trapped in the skin the quality and health of the skin will suffer. It is always a good idea to clean your face before exercising, as sweat can block pores and cause breakouts. Working in air-conditioned offices can also take its toll, although a plug-in ioniser will help to counteract the pollution and bowls of water placed around the office will add essential moisture to the air.

Alcohol has a dehydrating effect on the skin: excessive alcohol consumption results in dull, dry, irritated and blotchy skin. Emotional stress causes protein production that in turn triggers the immune system's white blood cells to clog the walls of blood vessels. This can result in sensitivity, redness and irritation that can lead to skin-related illnesses such as psoriasis, hives, eczema, rosacea and acne. In times of stress blood is directed to the major organs resulting in a pale, ashen look with its accompanying under-eye circles. Chronic stress slows skin cell turnover and causes a build up of metabolic toxins, making skin look sallow. Adrenal stress hormones also cause pimples. Fast track solutions to a clearer, more vibrant skin include reducing stress levels, getting more sleep and eating well.

skincare routine

Cleansing is the single most important thing that you can do for your skin. Your skin type will specify the type of cleansing required. Remember that your skin changes throughout the year and in different climatic conditions, which means that you will need to vary your skincare routine accordingly, particularly when travelling.

NORMAL SKIN is generally smooth, supple and velvety to the touch, with little sign of open pores. Skin colour is usually even and the skin typically has a healthy, radiant glow. Regular cleansing, toning and moisturising with periodic exfoliation and deep cleansing will help maintain the quality of the skin.

COMBINATION SKIN feels slightly thick, pores are open around the T-zone (forehead, nose and chin) where the skin is also shiny, and make-up has a tendency to disappear into the skin. Moisturise the dry areas more thoroughly and cleanse the oilier areas more carefully.

OILY SKIN comes with enlarged pores and an oily scalp. Smoother in texture, thicker and more pliable than other types of skin, oily skin maintains its elasticity and youthfulness for longer, which leads to fewer wrinkles. However, the sebum that helps to keep the skin from heavy wrinkling can lead to blackheads and skin breakouts. Regular cleansing is most important for this skin type.

DRY SKIN has a dull, matte texture and tends to flake and look white or grey in patches. It is often aggravated because the sebaceous glands are under-active or the skin has been exposed to the harsh elements of sun, wind, sea and central heating. Dry skin develops wrinkles and fine lines early and the dryness tends to intensify with age. The skin can appear red and blotchy as it tends to be thinner and can show expanded capillaries and blemishes from sensitivity. Eruptions, when they do appear, are normally in the form of whiteheads.

PROBLEM SKIN often suffers from blackheads, a mixture of secretions, old skin cells, keratin and melanin. An ayurvedic trick for keeping them at bay is to rub a wedge of red tomato over the face for five minutes and rinse it off. Tomato is rich in vitamins A, B, C and E and contains amino acids and salts such as lycopene, which make it a good skin astringent, but it should be used with caution by those with dry or sensitive skins.

Steaming is the most effective way of removing blackheads as they are brought to the surface and then can be eased out with tissue-clad fingers or by using special extractors. To steam your face pour boiling water into a bowl then add herbs such as lavender or a couple of appropriate essential oils from the list on pages 152–153. Jasmine has anti-bacterial properties and adds a delightful fragrance, while basil leaves are antiseptic and help clear blemishes.

Make a tent over your head and the bowl with a thick towel, lean over the bowl and let your face luxuriate in the warmth of the steam for about ten minutes. Take care not to over-steam as this can encourage the development of permanently open pores. Finish with a toner to seal pores, refine and rejuvenate.

cleansers

Once you have determined your skin type you can choose the most suitable cleanser: the drier your skin is the thicker the cleanser you will need. Cream cleansers are great for dry skins as they leave a light moisturising film over the surface of the skin. Wash-off gel cleansers are good for normal skins as they leave no residue, and foaming cleansers, which dissolve any surface oil, are perfect for oily skins. Regular soap is not the answer as it leaves alkaline residues that are very difficult to rinse off and can interfere with moisturisers.

Thoroughly cleanse your face before bedtime. Cleanse from the hairline to the base of the neck, massaging it in gently with circular movements and allow a minute or so for make-up to melt into it before removing. The decision whether or not to cleanse again in the morning is dependent on evidence of shininess or oil build-up over-night – sometimes a simple wipe with a warm, wet washcloth will suffice.

enhance

toners Popular due to the 'clean' sensation of freshness that they impart, toners can be used as part of a regular skincare routine as long as they contain no alcohol. Astringents are usually alcohol based and are too harsh for most skin types.

moisturisers Skin becomes dry and flaky if it does not get enough natural oil. Moisturisers are designed to correct any imbalance, act as a barrier against external elements and an occlusive barrier to hold in moisture. Choose one formulated for your specific skin type.

facial scrubs Scrubs slough off dull surface skin cells to reveal shiny new ones underneath and should be used in moderation – no more than once a week. Look out for scrubs with tiny smoothly rounded granules that are much gentler on the skin.

face masks Masks can be used as a weekly treat. For oilier skins look out for deep-cleansing ingredients such as kaolin, bentonite and zinc oxide; for drier skins that need moisture try milk protein, collagen, panthenol, water, azulene, chamomile, honey, hyaluronic acid and algae. Apply the mask thickly and only leave on for the recommended time.

facials Few sybaritic pleasures compare with a good facial. A facial provides the type of deep cleansing and massage that you can't do at home, with proper skin analysis.

Although they are not cheap, facials should be regarded as monthly preventative treatments. Shop around until you find a facialist who strikes the perfect balance between deep cleansing and de-stressing – remember you should leave a facial feeling relaxed and looking radiant.

Skin is thoroughly cleansed, scrubbed, steamed to warm and open the pores in preparation for extraction, massaged and then a mask is applied. Finally the skin is re-hydrated with moisturiser or protective cream. After-care instructions should be heeded as they are being issued by an expert who has spent the best part of an hour solely focused on the health and wellbeing of your skin.

facial oils Daytime skincare should be all about protection whereas at night skin needs to regenerate and rest. Treatment oils and creams are often prescribed to repair any damage done during the day. Oils penetrate more deeply into the skin than creams and when coupled with essential oils the brain is stimulated and soothed by the aromas. For a nourishing night-time treat try mixing 10ml carrier oil with no more than 8 drops in total of either a single essential oil, or a combination of up to four different essential oils, according to your skin's needs (see pages 152–153 for recommended oils).

When shopping for skincare preparations generally what you pay for is what you get. Always try to buy the best-quality ingredients you can afford, as quality is a measure of efficacy particularly when it comes to essential oils. Some of the most commonly found skincare terms and ingredients are listed in Inspire (see pages 152–153).

Do check the ingredients of every beauty item you buy to make sure that it will be suitable for your skin. The best aromatherapy and plant-based products tend to originate in Europe and Australia, whereas many cutting-edge high-tech solutions are discovered in the United States and Japan.

Pay attention to some of the smaller skincare companies who offer unique solutions for specialist areas in the marketplace – many of these have evolved in response to personal skin problems and offer proven solutions.

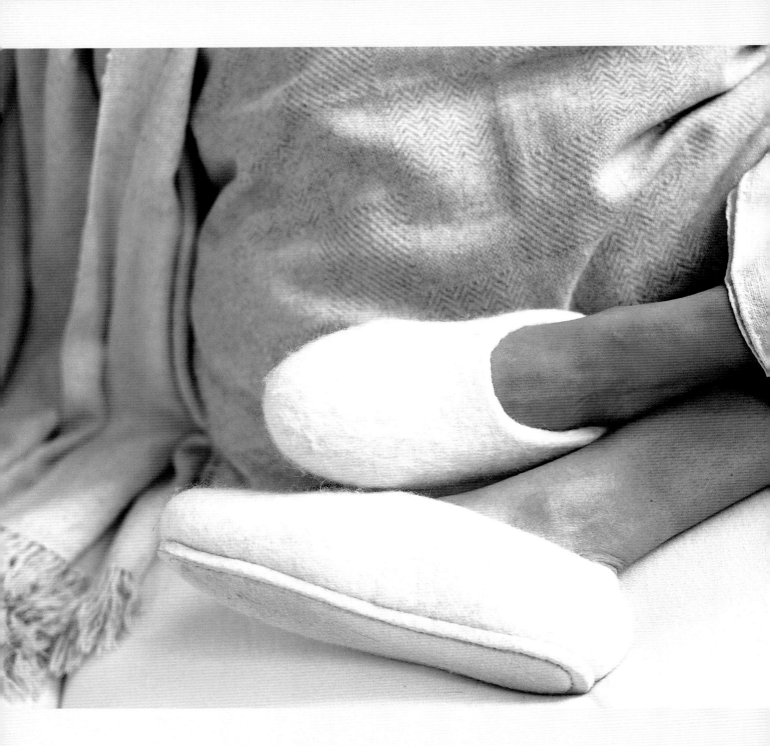

blissful body

Ask a man what he loves most about his partner and he may well say her soft, smooth skin. And he isn't talking about the skin on her face. It may be that the only time you really give your body a treat is before an important date or event, but why not treat yourself all the time?

skin-firming milk bath

skin-firming milk bath For most women today a bath too often means a quick shower to get clean but there is much more to a bath than that; it should be seen as a chance to relax and be pampered. The very words 'milk bath' conjures up images of Cleopatra bathing in asses milk, which might not be altogether appealing; however, the milk proteins in the contemporary version can render skin satiny smooth and glowing without any stickiness or unwelcome odour.

TO PREPARE AND USE THE BATH

1 heaped tablespoon milk powder
or
1 cup fresh milk
1 teaspoon oatmeal

Mix the milk or milk powder and oatmeal into a warm bath, then lie back and relax for twenty minutes. Using a warm, fluffy towel gently pat the skin dry. Beginning at the feet and working upward apply a moisturising body lotion to the skin.

If you would rather shower than bathe you can still benefit from the glorious effects of milk. In a bowl mix a cupful of milk powder with enough water to make a thick paste; apply to the skin and leave to work its magic for ten minutes, then shower off to reveal baby-soft skin.

oatmeal body scrub

oatmeal body scrub This is a gently abrasive firming scrub for when the skin is looking especially sallow after a long winter of being wrapped up against the cold.

TO PREPARE AND USE THE SCRUB

2 tablespoons oatmeal
water or milk (amount as required)

Mix together the oatmeal and enough water or milk to form a paste.

Take a handful of the mixture and gently scrub the body in circular movements, from the feet upwards, concentrating particularly on any areas of bumpy skin.

After a total of five minutes gently rinse off under a warm shower.

While the skin is still damp massage the following customised oil blend all over your body for luxuriously scented, satiny skin:

30ml skin-calming jojoba-based oil
4 drops petitgrain essential oil
3 drops each chamomile and jasmine essential oils

heavenly hands

In Sanskrit the hand is called HASTA, which means 'that through which we experience'. In fact, touch is one of the most important ways in which we show affection and love to others – think of parents holding their children's hand, the embrace of lovers and the tactility of friends.

Our hands never lie; they are one of the first parts of the body to show signs of ageing. Hand cream should always be applied after washing and nothing silkens paws quite like applying an ultra-rich hand cream at bedtime and wearing cotton gloves over the top while you sleep. A wonderfully simple and effective hand wash can be made, following the lead of restaurants the world over, by adding lemon slices to a bowl of warm water: acidic and fragrant lemon removes stains and banishes oil and aromas to leave the hands fresh and clean. Once a month treat your hands to a home-made hand scrub: mix lemon juice, crushed almonds and honey into a paste; gently rub your hands together for a few minutes; rinse thoroughly under warm water and pat dry.

Beautifully shaped nails of even length add grace to the hands. Nails are made of keratin, which when abused is liable to split and break; keep nails short if you want them to be stronger. Brittle nails can be treated with an increased intake of calcium-rich foods. For intensive treatment, take a calcium tablet before going to bed: this will not only strengthen the nails but, being a mild tranquilliser, will also help you fall asleep. Harsh chemicals dry out the nails and make them brittle, so use acetone-free nail-varnish removers and, wherever possible, formaldehyde-, toluene- and camphor-free nail polishes. White spots on the nails are indications of a zinc deficiency, so try to eat more seafood, particularly oysters.

Manicures are the best way to keep your hands soft and in shape and they also improve the circulation. A salon manicure is a worthwhile investment, as it will really help to get your nails in tip-top condition and encourage you to keep up the good work at home afterwards.

home manicure

Fill a shallow bowl with warm water and add a little mild shampoo or, better still, fragrant bath oil. Remove any nail polish with an acetone-free remover.

Starting with the little finger and working in, file the nails gently in one direction using a finely ground nail file – cutting can weaken the nails and may cause them to split. The nail should have a slightly rounded tip as square nails have a tendency to break.

Massage cuticle-softening cream into the cuticles and soak the hands in the prepared bowl of warm water. Gently pat the hands dry and carefully push back the cuticles, using the tip of an orange stick wrapped in cotton wool or the rubber end of a hoof stick.

Dip a nail-brush in the warm water and clean the nails. Rinse and dry the hands then massage for five minutes using a moisturising hand cream.

Soak a cotton pad in polish remover and gently wipe down all nail surfaces to be painted so every last vestige of hand cream has been removed.

Using smooth, even strokes from the base of the nail to the tip, apply a protective base coat followed by two coats of your selected polish. Finish with a topcoat to seal the varnish and extend the life of the manicure.

If you prefer not to use varnish then buff your nails for a pearly gleam.

enhance

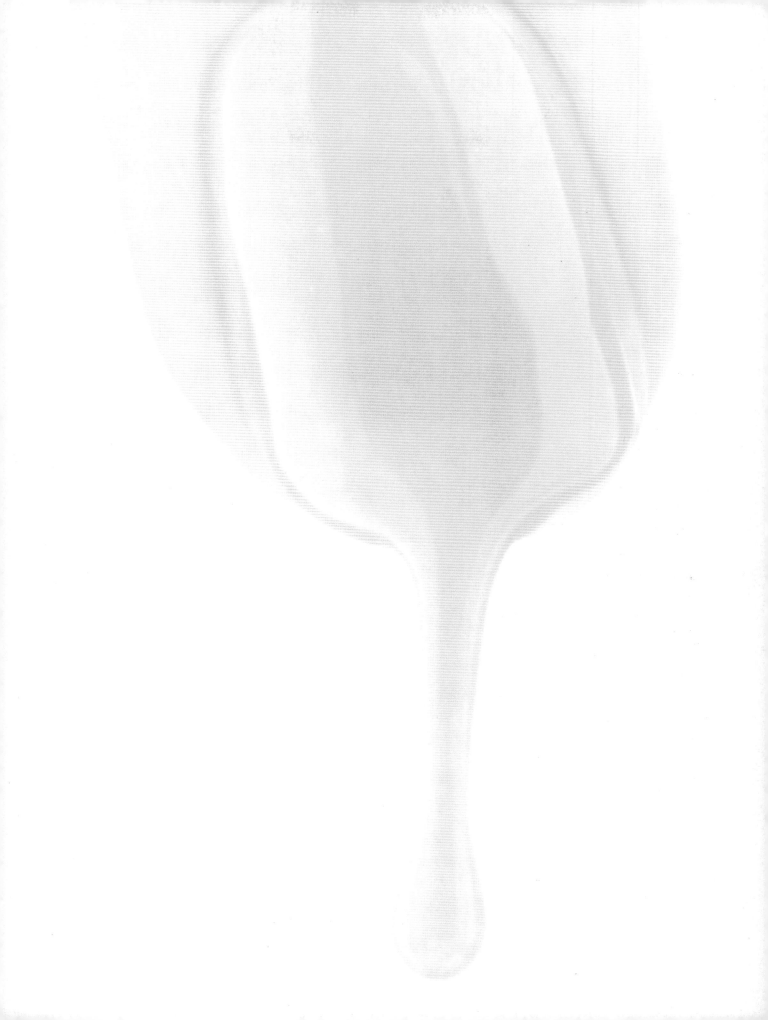

pampered feet

The Sanskrit word for foot is PADA, which means 'the point of contact with the earth' and 'that which is a source of nourishment to the physical body'. Feet often get neglected because they are under wraps for the greater part of the year. A regular pedicure is not simply a beauty indulgence but a necessity for foot health. A pedicure should be preceded with a few exercises: point your toes then flex your feet; rotate the foot from the ankle, first clockwise then anti-clockwise; pull each toe gently, then squeeze toes together with your hand.

home pedicure

Remove all traces of nail polish and soak your feet in warm, soapy water for ten minutes while relaxing. Add a little fragrant bath oil or a few drops of essential oil to stimulate the senses – peppermint cools, lavender heals and disinfects and chamomile soothes.

Clip any long toenails straight across to avoid in-growing nails and then file to even out any rough edges. Slough off dead skin with a pumice or foot exfoliating scrub, paying particular attention to the heels and soles.

Dry your feet thoroughly and use a foot file on any remaining areas of hard skin. It is very important to use this only on dry feet or you may file too deeply. Soak feet again and buff with a rough skin mouse.

Remove any dirt from under and around the nails with an orange stick and brush the whole foot gently with a foot brush. Apply cuticle cream around the toenails and massage well.

Soak the feet again for a further couple of minutes then dry the feet with a warm, soft towel taking particular care between the toes. Gently push back the cuticles with the tip of an orange stick wrapped in cotton wool.

Wipe the nails, apply a foot cream and massage well for about five minutes, using sweeping movements from the toes to the ankles. Soak a cotton pad in nail-polish remover then gently wipe down all nail surfaces to be painted to remove any remaining foot cream.

Separate the toes by winding a rolled tissue between them or using toe separators – this reduces the chances of smudging the varnish while it is drying.

Using smooth, even strokes from the base of the nail to the tip, apply a base coat to protect your nails, followed by two coats of your selected polish. Finish with a protective topcoat to seal the varnish.

Remember, depending on climatic conditions nail polish on toes can take up to one hour to dry. Applying a tiny drop of jojoba oil to each nail will help the polish set.

If you have your toenails polished in a nail bar or salon, take flip-flops along and wear them afterwards. If you rush your departure you may end up with the imprint of your tights imbedded in your new pedicure – in this worst-case scenario matters can usually be salvaged by the adept application of a further topcoat.

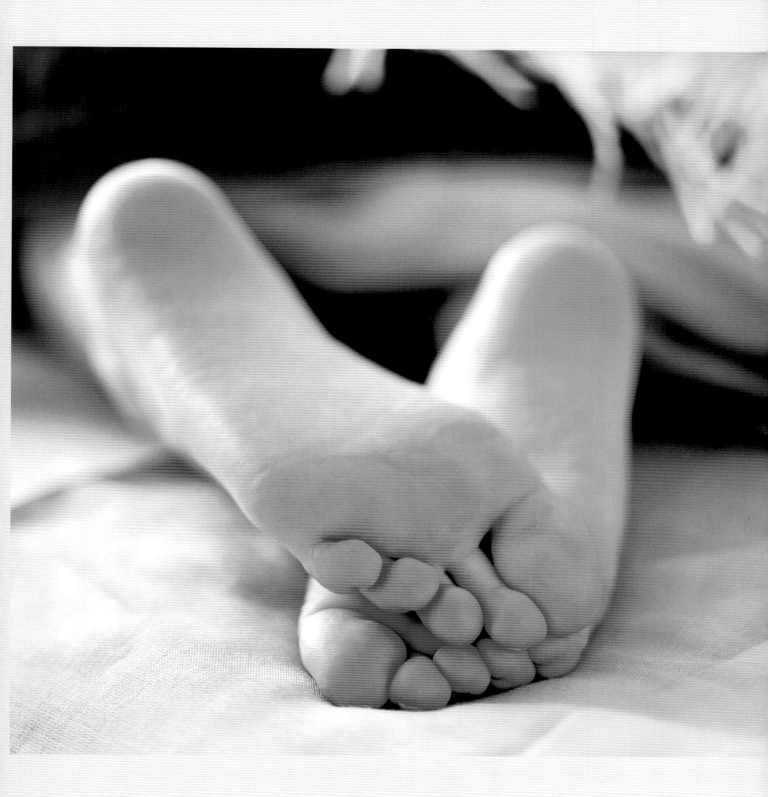

enhance

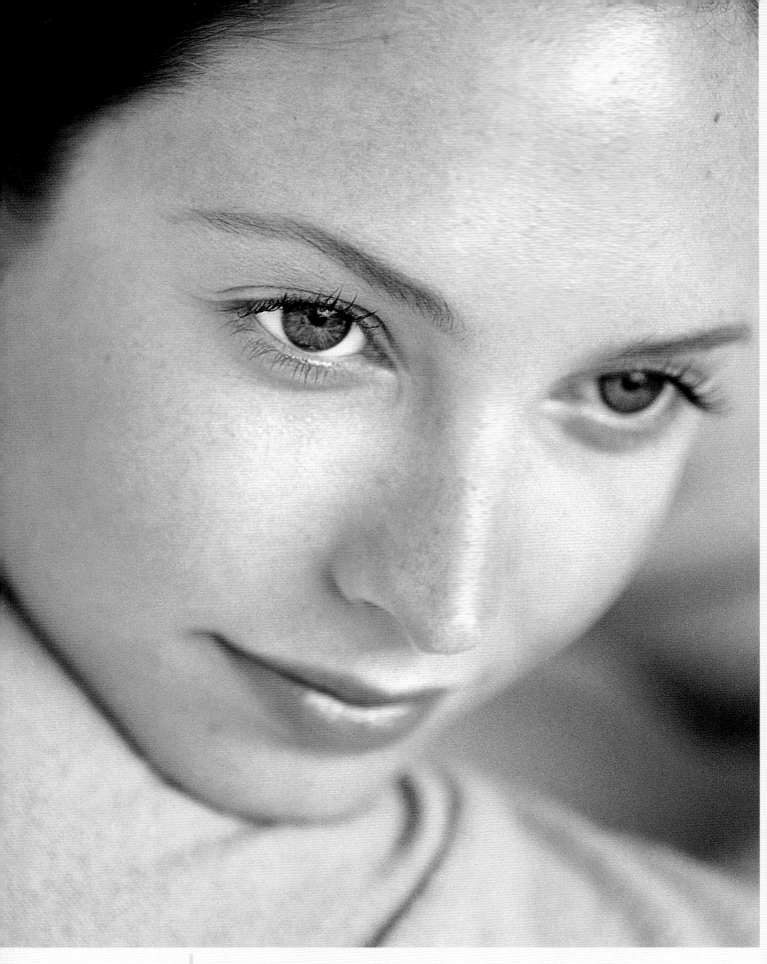

enhance

everyday make-up

As a canvas is to a painting, so the skin provides the perfect backdrop on which to highlight the eyes and mouth; good cleansing, toning and moisturising set the stage for the world of illusion that will follow. Remember that it's always more effective to enhance your good points than to heavily disguise any flaws.

foundation

Use foundation sparingly just where it is needed – under eyes, around the nose and mouth and over any blemishes – for even-toned, flawless skin. A light veneer looks radiant; when skin has a slight sheen it looks younger, as the naturally smooth surface of young skin reflects light. Look for a skin-illuminating base that can be worn under or mixed in with foundation. Change the foundation you use according to season: try a tinted moisturiser with SPF of at least 15 in the summer and a paler, more hydrating foundation in the winter. If your tinted moisturiser does not offer sun protection, put on a sunscreen first and wait at least five minutes for it to be absorbed before applying the tinted moisturiser. Experiment by mixing tinted moisturisers with your foundation to create a heavier base if you like more coverage in the summer.

Foundations are generally treatment-based so ensure you select one that is appropriate for your skin type and needs. Go with a foundation that is as sheer as you can get away with – less is more. It should blend with the colour of your neck not your face, so test it on the inside of a forearm in natural light – if necessary go outside the store – before purchasing.

Use a specially-formulated skin primer before you apply foundation to keep the skin from changing tone or looking mottled as the day goes on. Using fingers or a latex-free make-up sponge (dry gives more coverage, damp for a sheerer look) work with downward strokes, following the direction of any facial hairs lie, to render a smoother finish. The three key words for applying foundation are 'blend, blend, blend', especially around the nose, hairline and jaw line. Try to avoid using foundation under the outer corners of the eyes as it emphasises lines.

concealer

The eternal debate rages as to whether concealer should be used before or after foundation; I favour the latter as the application of foundation can easily rub concealer off. Using a concealer brush apply concealer around the nose, under the eyes and on the bone at the inner corner of the eyes. For a more natural cover-up on under-eye circles it is best to use a creamy concealer or brush on a blend of concealer and eye cream. Using a clean soft eye-shadow brush, set concealer with a light dusting of translucent loose power.

blusher

The one item of make-up that will give an instant healthy glow, blusher can also be the hardest to apply properly: the darker your colouring the more blush you need, but you should always aim for a natural, soft glow rather than trying to make a feature of your cheek-bones, which doesn't work. Match the tone of your blusher to your lipstick – warm or cool according to your look – and apply over foundation but under face powder using a proper blush brush (see page 57). For the most natural look smile into the mirror and apply to the apples of your cheeks when you are smiling and blend back a little towards the cheekbone. If you have dry skin it is best to use a cream blusher; gel blusher offers the sheerest form of coverage but should be applied over moisturiser not foundation to ensure good slip and even coverage.

Bronzing powder offers a natural, sun-kissed look for summer when dusted across the forehead, cheekbones, nose and chin. Shimmery bronzers look better on younger skins; for a more natural look use a matte shade that is neither too dark nor too orange.

face powder

To seal your look use a big, soft powder brush and loose powder. Use lightweight, translucent, light-reflecting powder rather than tinted powder as it allows an even coverage without adding colour. Blow away any excess powder on the brush before dusting your face and blend well to eliminate any powdery patches. Carry a compact of pressed powder with you, or better still some oil-blotting papers, to revive and re-set your make-up during the day.

alluring eyes

Health and happiness radiate through the eyes so they can be one of the first areas in which problems show. Dark circles can be triggered by lack of sleep and pollution; puffiness can indicate allergies and sensitivity towards products, or a diet too high in salt or alcohol. Never allow yourself to go to sleep still wearing eye make-up as the eyes and their surrounding area are very sensitive and neglect will soon start to show.

For a calming remedy for eyestrain soak cotton-wool pads in cool rosewater or cornflower water, place on closed eyelids then lie back and relax for 10–15 minutes. For a instant sparkle place still-warm tea bags over the eyes to utilise the excellent stimulating properties of tannin.

eyebrow shaping

As the archway to the eyes, eyebrows should always be well groomed. Shaping the eyebrows instantly tidies up the face and focuses attention on the eyes. To get the arch right, have your brows shaped by a professional. They can then more easily be maintained at home by plucking stragglers that fall beneath the defined curve. To determine the correct length for eyebrows hold a pencil against the outside of your nostril and align it to the inner corner of the eye on the same side – this point is where the brow should start. Swing the top of the pencil to the outer corner of the eye, so the pencil runs from the nostril to the eye – this is where the brow should end.

If you need to shape your eyebrows at home tweezing is the easiest method, but make sure you do it in natural light. Use stainless steel tweezers with slanted ends and a hand-held magnifying mirror. Thoroughly cleanse the area to be tweezed and make sure it is not greasy. Draw in the brow's natural line with an eyebrow pencil to act as a guide, then start plucking stray hairs one at a time. Always pluck hair out in the direction it grows and from under the brow to follow its natural shape. Work from the middle outward in both

directions; remember the highest part of the arch should be over the centre of your eye. After tweezing wipe the eye area with tea tree oil to prevent infection.

Threading, the most common method of facial hair removal in India, is becoming increasing popular here in the West. One end of cotton thread is held between the teeth while the middle of the thread is held in a taut loop with one hand while the other hand manoeuvres the other end of the thread. The mouth and hands work in a rhythm to catch the stray hairs within the loop and pluck them out with the movement of the thread.

Eyebrows are easiest defined using powder shadow in a shade just lighter than the brows. Apply in the direction of the hairs with a hard-edged angled eyebrow brush. This is easier than using an eyebrow pencil which often deposits hard, unnatural lines. Some make-up artists draw a line of concealer under the brow and blend this with a cotton bud to highlight and define the brow bone.

Brush your brows upwards and set with a coat of eyebrow gel to stop the brow hairs moving during the day; if you don't have gel use a touch of hairspray on an old toothbrush and lightly brush through the brows. If your eyebrows are long and straggly, brush them upwards and trim the ends slightly with a pair of nail scissors.

eyeliner

Eyeliner can be applied before or after eye shadow. For best results it should be used with a light hand: use a slanted or straight-edged eyeliner brush to smudge a dark powder eye-shadow lightly onto the top

enhance

54

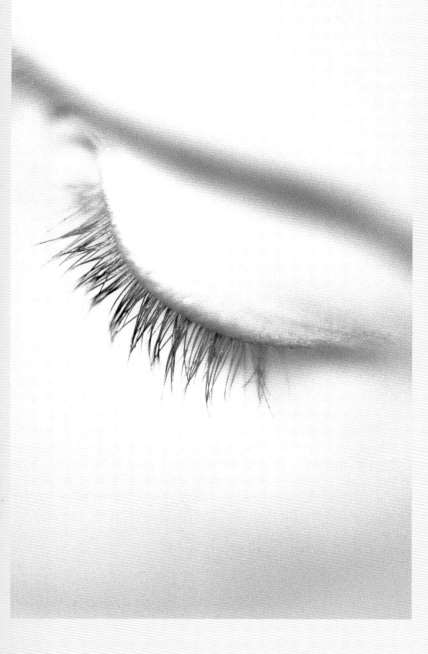

base is similar in texture to a light concealer and evens out the underlying skin tones while ensuring your eye shadow will stay fresh all day long. Use a neutral, highlighting shadow all over the brow and eyelid, then use a medium shade on the socket and edges of the eyes. Be wary of dark shades, which require an awful lot of blending to look good.

eyelash curlers

I truly believe in the often-maligned eyelash curler: if you buy good curlers with non-stick silicone pads your lashes will be gently curled rather than crimped. If you use a curler then do so before applying mascara.

For beautifully curled lashes begin on the upper lash roots, arranging the lashes between the two rims then gently squeezing the curlers for five seconds. Release and move the curlers towards the mid-lash region and repeat the process. Never pull the eyelashes with the curler clamped shut. Clean the curlers regularly with some cotton wool dipped in alcohol and make sure you replace the pad as soon as the rubber starts to crack.

mascara

Mascara thickens eyelashes and, depending on the design and quality of the brush, can also lengthen and separate them. Find a colour that suits your colouring to maintain the illusion of natural beauty: taupe or brown mascara looks far more natural than black on those with blond eyelashes. Apply several thin coats of mascara, separating the lashes as you go to avoid unsightly clumps. The easiest way to apply mascara is by looking down into a mirror and gently lifting the top eyelid. Sweep down the top of the upper lashes then sweep up from their underside to open the eyes, taking care to coat the shorter lashes at the corner of the eyes. For a more glamorous evening look apply mascara to the lashes of the lower lid, but only at the outer edges.

lashes; use a damp brush to get a deeper finish. If you prefer to use a pencil make sure it is sharp and that you smudge the line for a more natural look. Liquid liner can be used for a more dramatic look, but must be applied very carefully as it does not blend or diffuse. Lining just the top lashes defines and opens up the eye. Another way to open up the eye is to line the lower rims with skin-tone pink or white eyeliner. Work the eyeliner into the roots of your lashes to make them appear longer and thicker.

eye shadow

As the day wears on, eye shadow has a tendency to disappear, so try applying an eye-shadow base over the entire eyelid, blending up onto the brow bone, before applying eye shadow. This

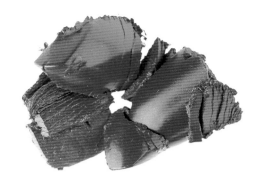

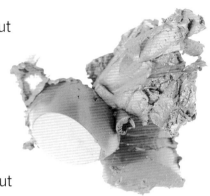

irresistible lips

One of the most alluring features of a woman is her mouth – the shape, the texture and the pout all draw attention. Add a soft smile to this and it becomes even more attractive: a happy, relaxed and ready smile for everybody makes people want to be near them; even the most beautiful woman in the world will look unattractive if her mouth is tight with anxiety, jealousy or hate. A smile lifts the face in a heartbeat. For some women lipstick is an instant mood booster and can make them feel more positive about the world even on a tough day.

lipstick Lipstick colours, highlights and corrects the form of the lips. Learning to shape your lips with make-up takes practise – subtlety is the key because a too-perfect mouth will only look contrived. To make thin lips look larger, smooth foundation over the edges and set with a little translucent powder to stop lipstick bleeding and reduce feathering. Then, with a natural-coloured lip pencil, draw an outline just outside the natural line of the lips. The peaks on the top line can be emphasised a little along with the curves but leave the corners alone. Use a lighter colour of lipstick in the centre of the lips and add gloss, which opens the lips and draws attention to them.

To tone down full lips cover them with a light veneer of foundation, set with powder, then draw the lip line just inside the natural line stopping short of the corners. Fill in the colour in the middle using the same colour all over and steer clear of gloss, particularly on the upper lip.

Use a lip brush to apply lipstick so that less goes further. For lipstick that goes on evenly and lasts longer apply a layer of lip balm and allow it to soak in for five minutes. Blot any excess with a tissue and apply a

layer of lipstick. Blot this with a tissue to leave a stain on your lips, then repeat the process again and finally apply one last coat of lipstick without blotting. After applying your final coating of lipstick put your finger in your mouth, close your lips around it and pull your finger out – this removes any lipstick from inside your lips that could rub off on to the teeth.

Apply lip liner after lipstick as it will look less hard-edged: no-one wants the dreaded ring of lip liner showing half-way through the morning. You do not need a different lip liner to go with each lipstick colour. Use a maximum of two different, neutral lip liners – one the same tone as your natural lip colour and another two shades deeper. Try using a lip pencil to both outline and colour in your lips, as this avoids lipstick bleeding into any fine lines. Top with light gloss for a more natural look.

Look out for lipsticks that contain anti-ageing ingredients, vitamins A and E, moisturisers and sun filters. If you get chapped lips exfoliate them once a week – apply a thick layer of lip balm then buff them with a soft dry tooth-brush, wipe them clean with a warm moist facecloth and then reapply another protective layer of lip balm.

teeth Keeping your teeth healthy and bright and your breath fresh demands effort. Brush your teeth after every meal, floss regularly with disinfecting tea tree-infused dental floss and try to avoid letting citrus fruit linger in your mouth as the acid environment they create are the biggest cause of tooth decay. Stress, surprise, surprise, is another major contributor as it brings acid into the mouth, which is another good reason to work on its elimination.

'Whitening' toothpastes cannot whiten teeth, but they may clean more effectively and help remove existing stains, prevent other stains building up and polish teeth to make them look shinier and brighter. A six monthly hygienist's appointment ensures plaque and stains are regularly removed and that the teeth are well polished. Having amalgam fillings replaced with composite or porcelain fillings may help your general health as evidence shows that the neuro-toxic mercury released from the amalgam can lead to a wide range of illnesses, including headaches and allergies.

Try to breathe through your nose as breathing through the mouth dries out protective saliva and can lead to teeth and gum problems. A quick way to get rid of transitory odours caused by strong-smelling foods is to chew on cardamom, cloves, aniseed, fennel seeds, mint leaves, holy basil leaves, an apple, carrot or cucumber. All of these also aid digestion, which affects the breath directly.

make-up brushes Having the right brushes is key to perfect make-up application. Good-quality brushes are a long-term investment, which, given proper cleaning and care, should last many years.

Lip-brush shapes and hair are a matter of personal choice. I prefer a sable brush with a squared-off end as this enables me to draw a precise lip line. Others may prefer a more rounded, synthetic version. There is an on-going debate about retractable versus non-retractable; if you go for the cleaner, retractable option make sure that the head does not move too much within its casing.

Look for an all-over eye shadow brush with a gently rounded sable head for general base colour application – choose the size of head that you feel comfortable controlling. A contouring or crease brush is usually best made of blue squirrel and allows easy application and blending of eye shadow in the eye socket.

Eyeliner brushes come in many guises and they vary in form according to the kind of eyeliner you wish to apply. For liquid application use a very fine sable or synthetic pointed brush that is retractable so it will not dirty your make-up bag. For wet or dry powder application a stiff, flat, synthetic brush is best – look for one that allows you to press or wiggle on the eyeliner without the hairs along the tip of the brush splaying and leaving too thick a line. Performance of these brushes can easily be tested on the back of your hand prior to purchase.

Another essential brush is a medium-sized blush brush. The best are made from a blend of blue squirrel and super-fine goat hair. Look for a head shape that is gently rounded at the end but flattened along the sides as this allows precise blush application as well as being good for general blending.

A powder brush will, generally speaking, be your biggest make-up investment and you do get what you pay for. A blend of super-fine goat and pony hair is ideal and look for a carefully contoured head that picks up powder well but only deposits it where and when you want it to.

essential haircare

A head of shiny, well-maintained hair provides instant glamour. In Vedic times women washed their hair with aloe vera gel, hibiscus flower juice and other fragrant herbs, and then oiled it with coconut oil scented with jasmine, rose or sandalwood. They dried their hair over incense and the fragrance would linger for days scenting the air with the slightest movement. Indians have long been noted for the immaculate condition of their tresses and many still follow a special Sunday routine of oiling their hair all over and only washing it the following morning. Families have secret hair-oil recipes based on coconut oil, which is instantly cooling and recommended in ayurveda for stress or a headache, mixed with any number of different herbs.

Physical and emotional health is the first step to shiny hair – eating well, fresh air and exercise and sufficient sleep are all essentials, along with a reduction in stress levels. Stress causes the blood vessels that feed the hair follicles to constrict, reducing the levels of oxygen and nutrients that can reach the hair. It also affects the scalp muscles at the point where the hair grows out of the scalp and can, over time, lead to excessive hair loss. Levels of the hormone androgen, responsible for the thinning of hair in men, can increase and excessive sweat production will make the hair and scalp greasy. **A good protein diet that includes meat, fish, eggs, pulses and dairy products strengthens hair from the inside.** Vitamin B is absolutely essential and the best source of this is brewer's yeast – one capsule a day should improve the condition dramatically. Iodine helps boost the circulation to the scalp so eat plenty of fresh seafood.

Hair is made up of overlapping layers of keratin, which can stretch up to 30 per cent in length, swell up to 14 per cent in diameter and absorb its own weight in water. When the protein bonds are altered, through perming or colouring, hair becomes more susceptible to breakage. When the layers lie flat and smooth, each strand reflects light making it shine. We are born with between 150,000 and 200,00 hair follicles, with redheads having the least and blondes the most. We lose between 40 and 100 hairs a day naturally and hair grows on average half an inch a month (faster in summer than winter). The hair shaft consists of three layers: the medulla or spongy central core; the cortex or surrounding central fibres, which make up the bulk of the hair; and the cuticle or over-lapping outer layers of the cells. Hair thickness is determined by the size of the dermal papilla that can change through illness and hormonal fluctuation.

enhance

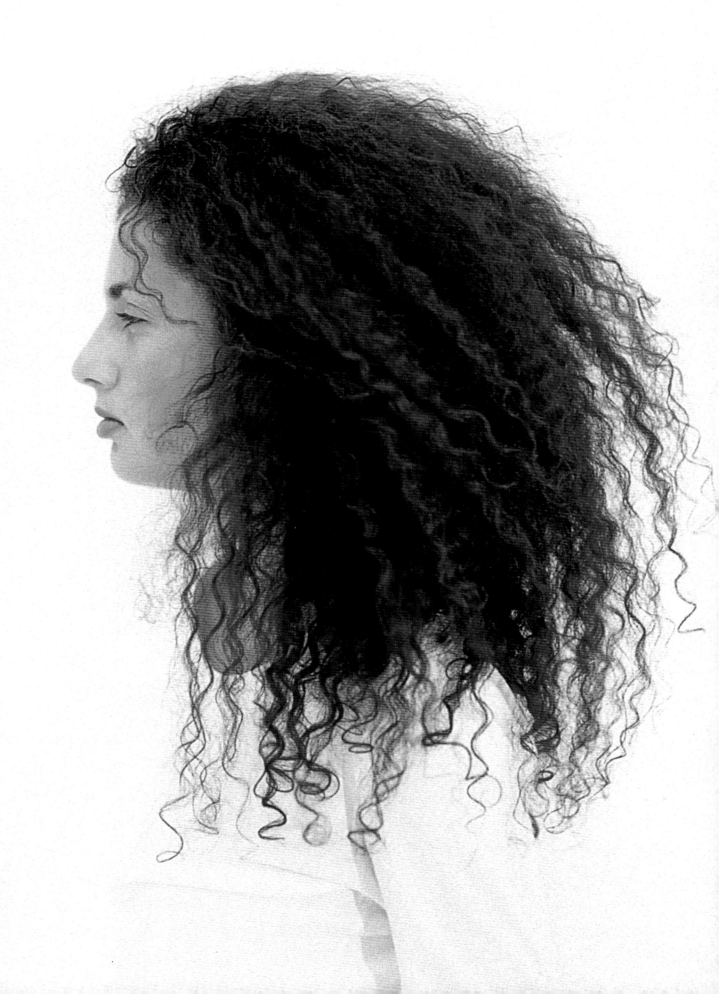

enhance

anti-dandruff rinse A quick way to control dandruff is to rinse hair after shampooing with a tablespoon of cider vinegar in a cup of water. To check excessive oil secretions and give a gentle exfoliation massage fresh apple juice, a mild acid, into the scalp. A relaxing scalp massage with warm olive oil can also clear up occasional bouts of scurfiness as well as help prevent hair loss. Dry massaging the scalp with the fingertips for twenty minutes every week is extremely beneficial as the movement improves the circulation and encourages the sebaceous glands to secrete oil.

shine-enhancing rinse Try a final rinse of lemon juice, beer or vinegar. The acid they contain removes any final traces of shampoo or conditioner and smoothes down the hair cuticles. Wash your hairbrush regularly with warm water and a little shampoo; add a couple of drops of tea tree oil to act as a disinfectant.

To keep hair in fine condition you need to look after it properly. Wash only as necessary and condition the hair to keep it shiny. All traces of conditioner, unless formulated as a leave-on product, must be rinsed away or the residue will leave the hair lank and sticky. Apparently one in three people do not wet and rinse their hair in clean water, preferring to dunk back in the bath water. To work effectively modern haircare formulations require plenty of water to release conditioning agents and remove dirt. Hair should be washed anything between daily and twice a week, but if your hair is looking good do not change your routine. Hair does get used to some of the newer volumising products, so if you think your products are no longer performing as they used to switch for a while and then go back to the original product for better results.

The main constituents of shampoo are water, fragrance and surfactant or soap-less detergent. Lathering is purely cosmetic and has no correlation with efficacy. Preservatives are added to protect against contamination, thickening agents bolster texture and there may be other additives such as hydrolysed protein, which fills the gaps in the hair cuticle boosting shine and making hair appear thicker. Panthenol or pro-vitamin B5 is also often used as it penetrates the hair shaft and improves condition. Conditioners deposit a lubricant on the hair that reduces static and makes hair easier to style.

Dandruff describes myriad scalp conditions that lead to visible flaking. Skin cells shed all the time, but this process can be accelerated for a number of reasons: an increase in natural yeast, stress, using a shampoo with too high a surfactant content, or inadequate rinsing. When the scalp is dry, flakes appear light and powdery, whereas on an oily head they can clog together. Keeping all brushes and combs really clean is essential.

To improve hair shine, elasticity and strength try a weekly intensive hair-conditioning treatment. Any conditioning treatment benefits from the application of heat, as this opens the pores and allows for better absorption – after a workout why not apply an oil or mask to your hair and then relax in the sauna or steam room of the gym. To restore moisture to the hair and protect it from the sun, wind and free radicals, try applying a conditioning oil before your morning run. A little oil may remain after the hair is washed which will act as a protective coat through the day. A special detoxifying shampoo can be used once a week, to rid the hair of any build up. Even if you cannot leave oil on your hair for very long just cover your scalp with a plastic shower cap to keep the heat in for about twenty minutes. Make good use of this time by soaking yourself in a tub of warm, scented water.

Changing your hairstyle is the easiest and most dramatic way of reinventing yourself, but approach the idea with caution. Be logical about the style that you ask for – only occasionally does the season's fashionable cut coincide with what suits you. In the same

60

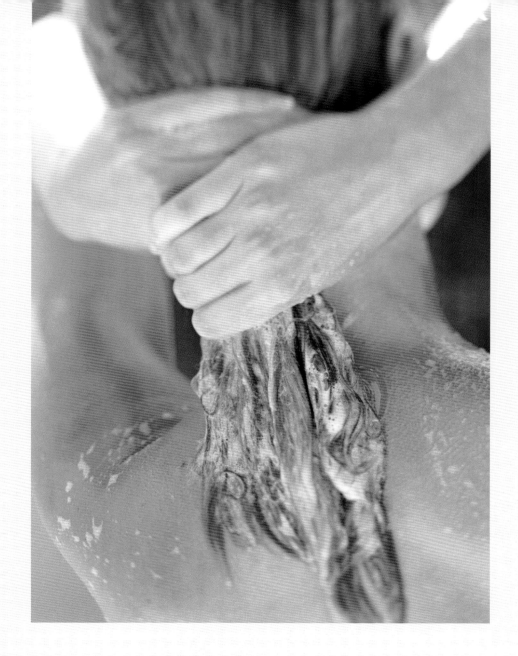

way, changing your hair colour is very easy but it is important to choose the right shade that flatters your skin tone and gives life to your whole face. Remember, **grey hair alone does not make a woman look old unless she behaves that way.** Any change in hair colour should be accompanied by a review of eye and lip make-up to complement your new shade. Seek objective, professional advice on changing your hairstyle or colour to enhance your features.

Invest in a good hairdryer – at least 1500watts with two air speeds, heat settings and ideally a cold button. **Overheating and over-processing are the two main reason for hair losing its shine** so do not start styling your hair until it is about 80% dry. Hair styling products are either oil- or water-based and are designed to increase or decrease the hair's tensile strength. Hair oils, serums, creams and pomades are meant to decrease volume, increase shine and smooth the hair. Sprays, gels and mousses are meant to increase volume. Sticks and waxes are used to add texture. Hair type determines which type of styling product is preferable.

enraptu

enrapture

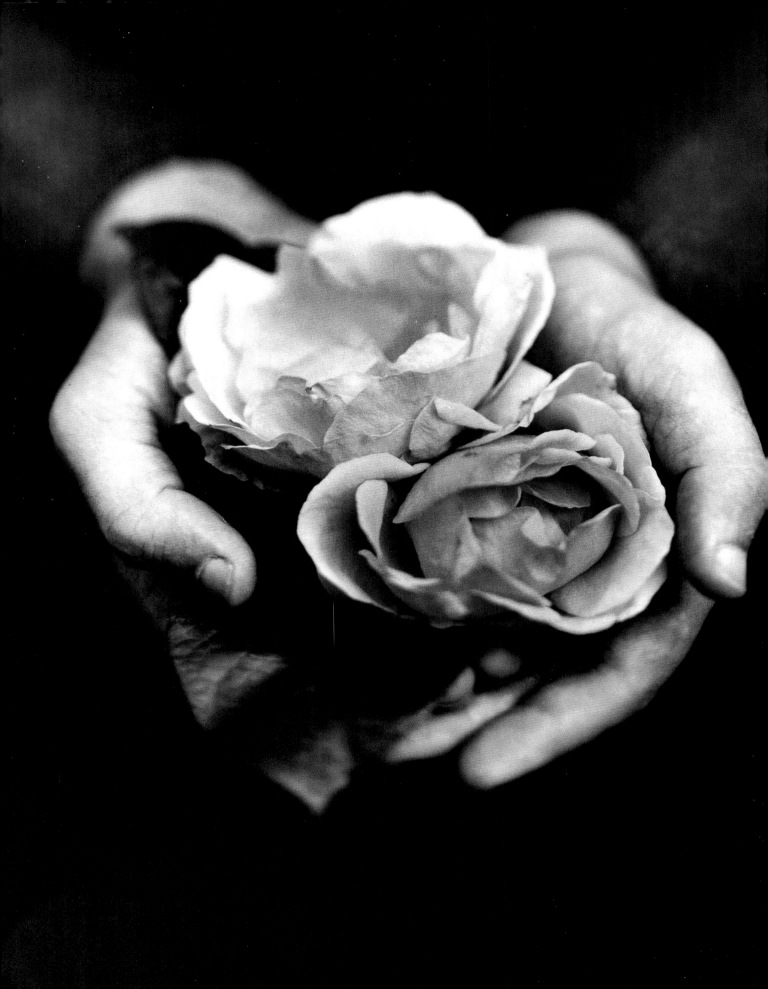

enrapture

There are times when we want to break out, throw moderation to the wind and indulge in hedonistic sensuality. Pampering ourselves can be truly inspirational, whether it takes the form of buying a new perfume, spending time on our make-up before an important date, indulging in the finer things in life for an evening or redecorating the entire home to enrich the senses. One thing is for certain: the efficacy of whichever route we take will be influenced by all five senses.

Our home is our castle, our refuge, our cocoon, and should nurture, inspire and delight us. The décor of our home should subtly stimulate the senses and produce an ambience in which we feel pampered all the time. When we discover the sensual feast that can be created with colour, texture, music and fragrance our homes and our lives will be enriched.

Fragrance is one of life's great pleasures. A potent means of personal expression, scent has the ability to trigger forgotten memories and emotions and to transport us to a different place in time. Aromas travel to the olfactory bulb, part of the brain's limbic system, which is associated with our basic emotions, memory, sexual feelings, learning and sense of smell. In the twenty-first century we are very conscious of how scent can be used to enhance our lives by using them to fragrance our bodies and our homes.

Natural essential oil scents carry an inherent code that affects the mind and body independently of what the brain associates with it: rosemary, eucalyptus and peppermint alleviate mental strain while vanilla, jasmine and chamomile will calm the mind, regardless of any associations stored in our memory. Essential oils offer a natural way to fragrance the home with nurturing, calming or welcoming aromas, scent the body with sensuous, romantic perfumes and stimulate or relax the mind during bathing routines.

Smell is also closely connected with taste, enhancing and clarifying flavours for a richer, fuller experience. For a true sense of decadence we can open a bottle of chilled champagne or wine, fill an elegant goblet and let our favourite tipple slip down while we lie relaxing in an aromatic bath. Whatever your favourite route to happiness, however you discover your personal pampering nirvana, remember that you are worthy of every minute you spend on yourself. Take pleasure in all your senses – be aware of all sights, scents, textures, sounds, tastes and feelings that surround you. Relax; enjoy; be aware that you deserve to be happy and content; feel loved.

indulgent interiors

The environment in which we live affects our mood and wellbeing dramatically. Use your favourite colours, fabrics, items and fragrances to create a home that is personal to you and in which you feel happy and at peace. Simple changes can make a significant impact on the feel of the home, from adding a small lamp or a few candles to create different light levels, to playing your favourite music softly while you lie back on luxurious, colourful floor cushions.

Colour has a subliminal influence on our mood: envisage the rich jewel tones of Morocco and India – spicy burnt oranges through scarlet reds, magenta pinks through deep midnight purples – which are colours that you can almost feel and taste. Red is the symbol of life, of strength and vitality. Orange, the colour of joy and happiness, symbolises feminine and creative energy. Magenta enables us to let go and flow with wherever life takes us – a bit daunting for our personality but bliss for the spirit. When magenta fades to pale pink it becomes the colour of spiritual love.

Take yourself to Asia and the Middle East for texture: opulent swathes of raw silk, deep-pile velvets and satins with gold and jewel-encrusted detail; hand-cut crystal chandeliers reflect a hundred candles in the balmy, fragrant air. In winter think of plush, faux-fur throws and sheep-skin rugs that you can sink your feet into when you climb out of your four-poster bed. For unbridled bed-time comfort, sheets are a choice between crisp linen, sensual silk or high-thread-count, rosewater-scented, Egyptian cotton, and the bed is resplendent with embroidered, beaded, goose-down pillows and bolsters.

If you already have the décor that you love, or you don't want to spend time painting and creating, change the ambience of your home by indulging a little every now and then. Whether you are getting into the mood for an important date or creating a sensory evening for yourself at home, it is important to pamper yourself with abandon once in a while.

Realise your dream of the perfect evening. Bowls of fragrant roses abound, the champagne is on ice and Charles Aznavour is crooning in the background while delicious vapours escape from under the bathroom door. Bathed in softly scented candlelight the claw-foot tub is scattered with rose petals, and luxurious foaming bath oil melts into the warmth of the water. The phone is off the hook, a filled champagne flute awaits, and you finally sink a manicured foot into the fragrant bath, feeling treasured and loved.

Music can lift our spirits when we feel down, carry us away on a romantic journey and inspire us when creativity is lost. For the perfect musical accompaniment to an evening of pure indulgence, play something that makes you blissfully happy, such as classic French love songs like *Un homme et une femme* by Nicole Croiselle and Pierre Barouh, beautiful and moving jazz like that of French chanteuse Liane Foley or, for a classic treat, lose yourself in the dulcet tones of Nat King Cole.

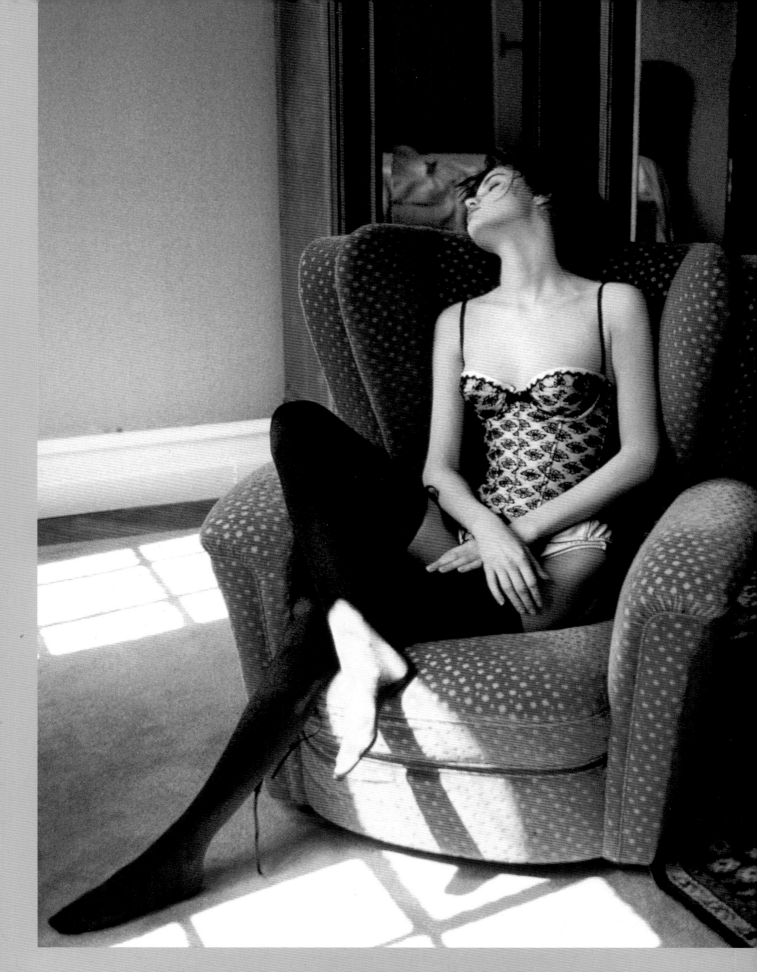

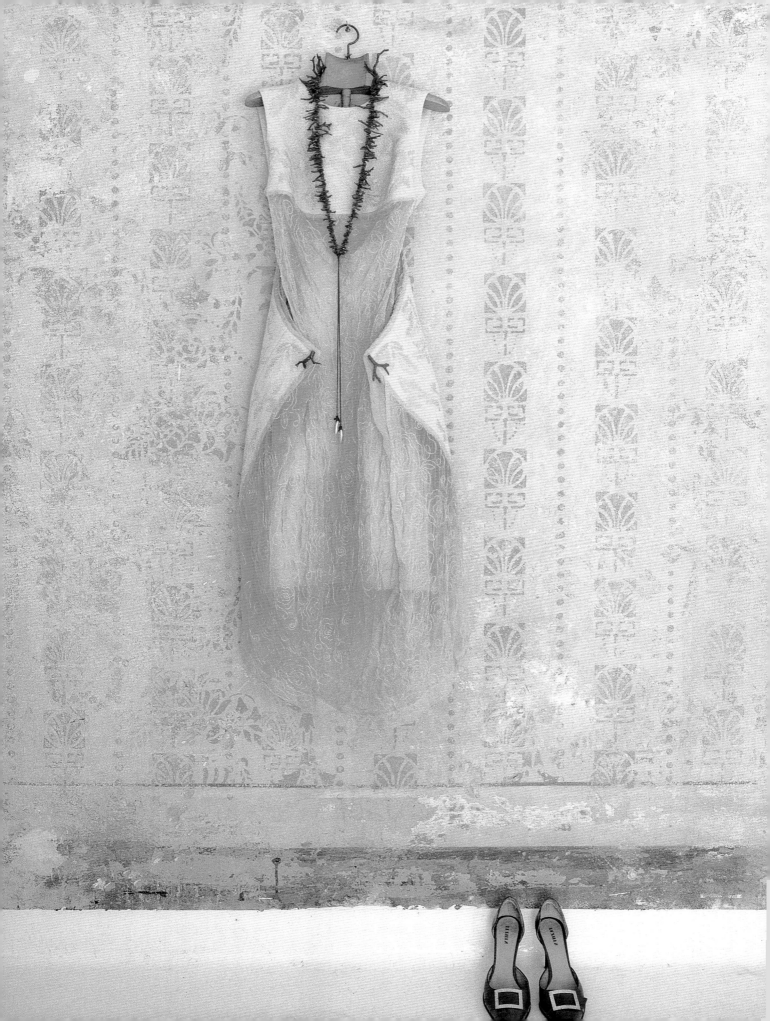

enrapture

ambient aromas

Fragrance has always been associated with sensual allure and an aura of mystery, so use it to create an ambience of indulgent relaxation. Earthy tuberose, creamy jasmine, warm amber, spicy frankincense and powdery fig leaf are all sensual fragrances that work well to create a heady, voluptuous atmosphere. Men are attracted by woody fragrances, such as cedar, sandalwood and fir balsam, particularly when combined with nutmeg, cinnamon or vanilla.

Scented candles can be a very effective way of filling a home with sensual aromas as they also offer a warm, flattering light. The best fragrances are usually found in poured candles that have a continuous burn time of between 10 and 50 hours. Candles are at their most romantic when used in groups of differing heights, but it may be best to mix scented and unscented candles so the fragrance is not overpowering.

The burning of incense is shrouded in many beliefs and customs but it has mostly been associated with practices of devotion; in China it is said that as the smoke spirals towards the heavens it acts as a portal through which humans and spirits connect. The most popular scents are oriental wood blends, with musk, rose and patchouli adding a touch of sensuality. Fragranced incense sticks and cones have come a long way from their hippy heritage. Top-quality, Japanese-manufactured incense is fast becoming a firm favourite with the travelling fashion cognoscenti who use it to create a more homely feel in anonymous hotel rooms.

Vaporising essential oils is a highly effective way of releasing their myriad properties. Place a little water in the well at the top of the vaporiser or oil burner then add 3 or 4 drops of the chosen oil or blend. Romantic oils include bergamot, jasmine, neroli, patchouli, rose and ylang ylang. Oils can also be added to a small bowl of hot water placed on top of a radiator. A beautifully simple way to surround yourself with the natural fragrance of essential oils is to create a household spray: add 2 drops of rose, neroli or lavender to 150ml of water, decant into a spray bottle and use to spritz your laundry and bedlinen before ironing.

In India the fragrance of the rose is favourite, followed by the kewra, or screw pine flower, and jasmine. Another highly prized scent is that of khus, a fragrant grass, which is woven into door curtains so each time someone passes through the gentle perfume is released. Another subtle way to bring elements of the natural world into your home to combine beauty and scent is to use cubes of solid amber resin. Place the amber inside a perforated, decorative perfume holder or mix into a spice- or wood-based pot pourri and enjoy its distinctive, warm Oriental fragrance.

aromatic indulgence

Personal fragrance and passion are irrevocably entwined – the ultimate sensory experience is also a highly sensual one. Fragrance has long been regarded as the most potent sense of seduction. Kama, the Hindu God of Love, carried flowers rather than arrows in his quiver whilst the Greek goddess Aphrodite dispensed beautiful aromas to aid seductions.

Among mere mortals there has always been the hope that a particular scent will make us irresistible to others. To this end, perfumers continue to try and exploit the aphrodisiac properties of specific scents from tuberose and jasmine to orange blossom and amber.

Since ancient times flower extracts and essences were widely used for bathing, hair and body anointing and to fragrance homes and temples. Indonesian royalty used to beautify themselves for ceremonious occasions with a series of cleansing treatments called a lulur bath. This would involve soaking in a fragrant tub filled with frangipani flowers, followed by a sea-salt exfoliation and a final, soothing yoghurt bath to soften the skin; silky smooth and subtly scented skin should inspire us all to take more time over bathing. By enhancing all our senses and allowing ourselves time to enjoy the experience, we not only cleanse our body but also lift our spirits.

Cleansing rituals can have a profound effect on how we feel both internally and externally. Bathing is an opportunity to incorporate aromatherapy in a very relaxing, comforting, womb-like environment. The combination of the water's soothing warmth and the effects of essential oils promote inner reflection and contemplation. Introducing essential oils into your daily routine can enhance your life considerably by promoting a positive mood or subtly altering a negative mood. Try building a library of essential oils with which to experiment (see pages 152–153 for ideas). The essential oils can be blended with carrier oils for facials, massages or baths, or used undiluted as burning oils to diffuse in the atmosphere. Create your own rituals for various moods and purposes: getting ready for a big night out, relaxing after a long day, relieving aches and pains or treating symptoms of ill health.

enrapture

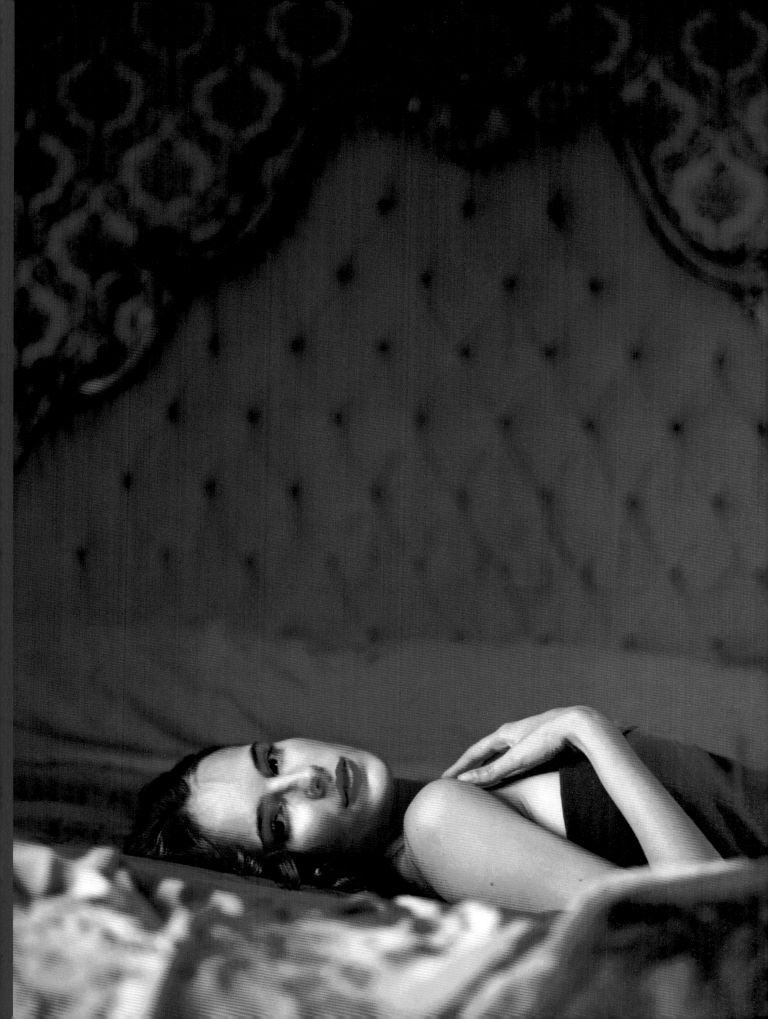

We seem to have an enduring fascination with how the body smells, but perfume alone is rarely a turn on; the scent of the body beneath the fragrance veil is the true aphrodisiac. We were not always so uncomfortable with this truth: Napoleon famously sent word to Josephine, 'I will be arriving in Paris tomorrow evening. Don't wash.' The body exudes a scent as personal as a face, which changes from time to time as its complex aromas vary with health, diet, emotion and age. Perfume should mingle with the body's own distinctive smell, heightening and enhancing it rather than masking it.

Remember that however many rare and costly ingredients go into the making of a perfume the final and most unique one will be added by your own skin. Body chemistry, the oils, minerals and moisture secreted by the glands beneath the skin's surface as well as the composition of your skin will make a particular fragrance smell different on you than on anyone else. Certain perfume essences are more seductive than others, but a scent that may smell voluptuous on one wearer can be earthy or fresh on another. Moreover when a fragrance is first applied, the individuality of your skin will make it smell different from how it smells in the bottle and different again in a little while when it has had a chance to warm up and further react with your skin. A perfume may smell heavenly one day and inconsequential the next. Context is everything.

perfume alone is rarely a turn on; the scent of the body beneath the fragrance veil is the true aphrodisiac

The appeal of fragrances can also change during the different seasons: lighter, citrus and white-floral, or chypre, fragrances are generally more appealing in warmer weather while sensuous, spicy Orientals come into their own during colder months. Aldehydic florals are favourites of women who want a modern yet sensual feeling from their fragrances, as the synthetic aldehydic notes add a champagne-like sparkle to the top notes. Sweet florals attract aficionados who are said to hide their passion, while strong, provocative women gravitate towards spicy, powdery chypres based on the contrast between bergamot top notes and mossy base notes. Oriental fragrances, made up of florientals and spicy orientals, are musky, spicy and voluptuous and tend to appeal to those who like to experience life in all its intensity.

Once you have found a fragrance you are attracted to try it on your body. Close your eyes and really smell it. Forget about the packaging and marketing hype; concentrate on the scent itself. The top note is the initial smell when you first open the bottle and spray it on your skin, and usually lasts about 15 minutes. The middle note or the heart of the perfume comes through after about 10 minutes exposure to the air and lasts for the next hour. Finally, the heavier base note slowly develops and lingers for several hours.

Where you put your fragrance can be as alluring as the fragrance itself. Coco Chanel was a proponent of fragrance being placed wherever you want to be kissed. The Greeks went as far as prescribing an aromatic oil for every body part: aphrodisiac rose was dabbed onto the neck, base of spine and the navel, breasts were massaged with thick, perfumed palm oil and feet were scented with warm, stimulating essences of sandalwood and clove. Fragranced feet were also popular in ancient Jerusalem where myrrh and balsam were placed in young women's shoes. The French favoured scented gloves and Japanese geishas originally infused their kimonos with fragrant incense, although Western fragrances are now also gracing their hair and necks. As a way of taking fragrance's sensual past into a contemporary context, lighter versions of perfumes are being made to mist into hair, and fragrant dusting powders are being used on the feet and lower back.

where you put your fragrance can be as alluring as the fragrance itself

The type of perfume used will inform how long its scent lasts on the skin. Regular, alcohol-based fragrances fade quite rapidly, depending on the concentration. Oil- or cream-based fragrances, however, have greater staying power. By using complimentary bath, body and perfume products, fragrance can be layered on the skin ensuring a subtle delicate aura that lasts throughout the day. The rule of taste, however, still applies: if you are wearing the right amount of perfume only you, and someone close enough to kiss you, should be able to catch the scent of it. Apply perfume discretely and modestly as, like all smells, perfume leaves a strong impression on the subconscious mind. A memory of a person or place will be often accompanied by that of an associated aroma; a recognised scent can lead your mind back to past events. The remembrance of a fragrance can keep a passion alive even if it fills the soul with regret for the passing of time.

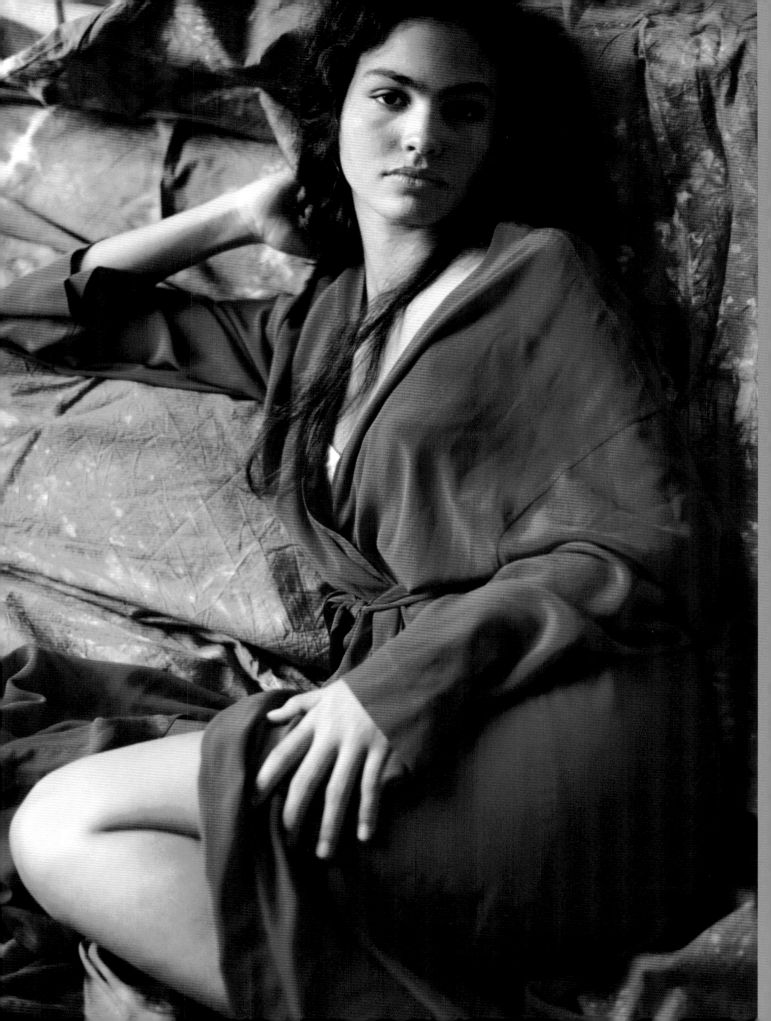

enrapture

sensual sanctuary Water has a hypnotic hold over us.

Water purifies and regenerates. Immersed in water the petty cares of the day drift away. Perfume heightens the aura of sanctuary by adding another sensory dimension to the bathing experience. Whilst luxuriating in a fragrant bath you automatically start to breathe more deeply, you become lost in thought, you lose track of time. In the tub we regress, recalling the womb, escaping the present as we lie back and relax. This fragrant aura stays with you for some time afterwards amplifying the sensual pleasure, a feeling that all things may be possible or that nothing needs to be done and that it may simply be enough for you.

romantic aromatic bath
This heart-warming bath will get you in the mood before an important date and will also help to increase the ardour of your loved one. It is uplifting and confidence boosting, the perfect way to treat yourself even when love is the last thing on your mind.

TO PREPARE AND USE THE BATH

Run yourself a warm bath and add the following customised oil blend:

4 drops heart-lifting rose essential oil
4 drops aphrodisiac ylang ylang essential oil
2 drops clarifying lemon essential oil
20ml sweet almond oil

Swirl the bath water round to disperse the oils. Lie back in the tub and breathe deeply for twenty minutes to allow the blend of aromas to lift your spirits and open your heart.

sensuous self-indulgence
Throw those cares away and plan an evening of pure self-indulgence. Sink into a wonderfully uplifting and relaxing bath to soothe your mind and pamper your body.

TO PREPARE AND USE THE BATH

Run yourself a warm bath and add the following customised oil blend:

4 drops de-stressing rose essential oil
4 drops tension-soothing sandalwood essential oil
1 drop stimulating juniper essential oil
20ml sweet almond oil

Swirl well in the water. Relax into the tub and let the oils gently work their magic.

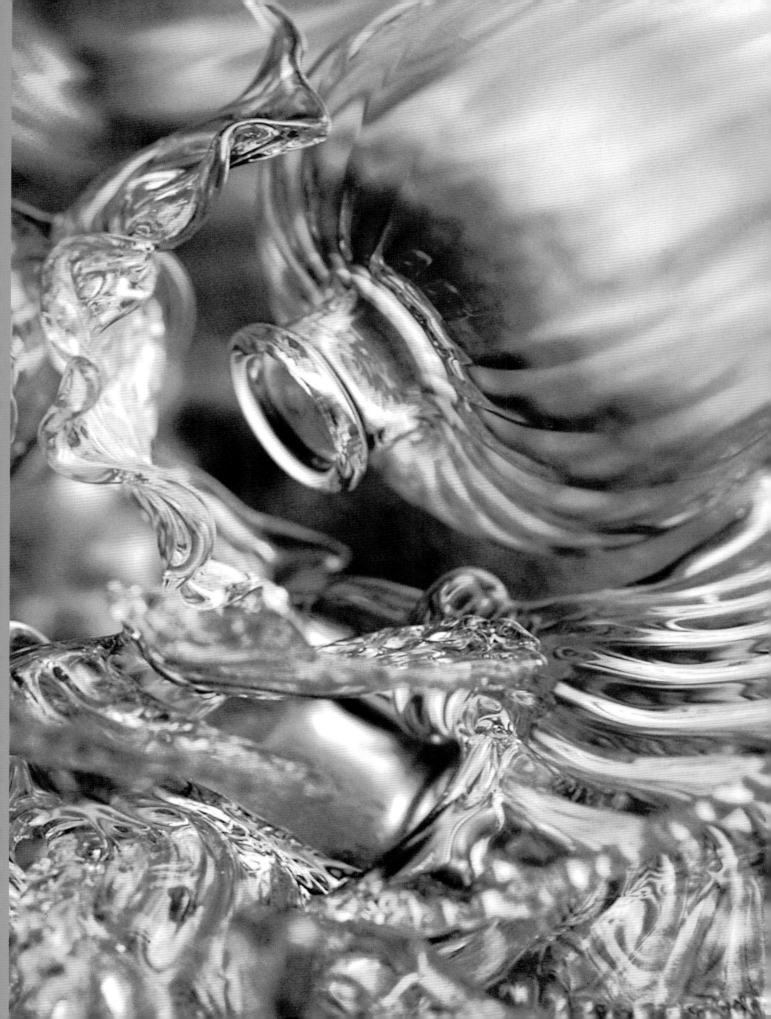

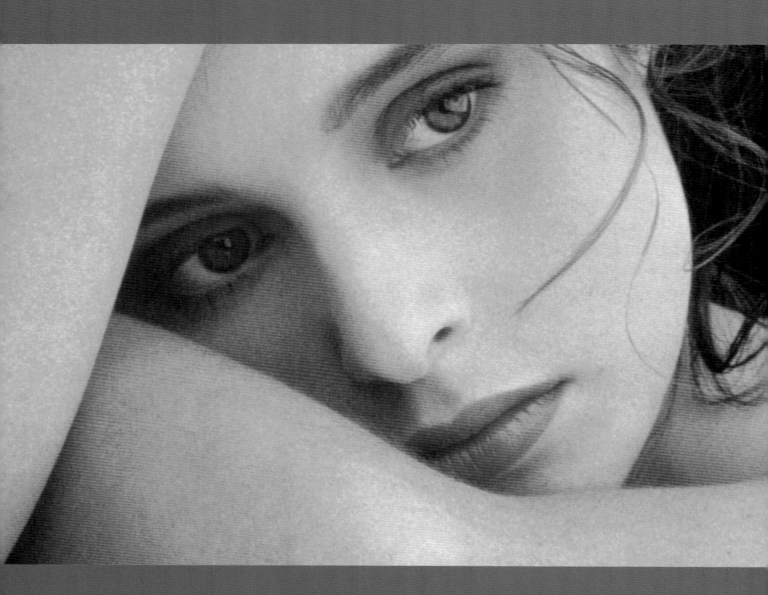

night-time make-up

Looking glamorous does not mean applying make-up with a trowel. The most common complaints about make-up from men are 'she wears too much', 'her make-up comes off on my clothes', and 'there's a visible line where her make-up ends and her skin begins'. The difference between evening and daytime make-up is in the colours rather than the application: use a foundation that gives a little more coverage, a lipstick that is deeper, richer or more shimmery, a pearly highlighter on your brow bone and darker colours on your eyes.

enrapture

Think about where you will be spending the evening and the possible light levels you may encounter. If the light will be low you may want to add a little definition around your eyes, but even if you won't be spending too much time in brighter light make sure you look natural and elegant rather than made-up. Consider your outfit and your hairstyle and how these might affect your make-up: if you have a special hair-style would you prefer to make a feature of your eyes and draw attention upwards, or do you want to highlight your new dress by using a glossy lipstick of a complementary colour? Whatever make-up you choose, always apply it with a light hand; less is more, even for the evening.

Use foundation, concealer and face powder in the same way that you would for the day. As there is no natural light to contend with at night you may choose a foundation that offers a little more coverage than the one you use in the daytime. If so, be extra careful when applying it: blend it in well and ensure that your face is the same colour as any exposed skin on your body.

For added night-time drama, subtle, creamy highlights work anywhere the skin would normally shine: sweep across the brow bone, the eyelids and the cheekbones; or add a touch of gloss to the middle of the bottom lip. If you want to add some shimmer to your evening look, remember that a highlighter can attract light so keep it away from any lines or blemishes. If your neck and chest are bare try sweeping a light bronzing powder over the entire area.

Smoky eyes work best in softer evening light. First cover the eyelid with a base of primer or concealer topped with some translucent powder, and then apply a black eyeliner pencil along the upper and lower lashes smudging in well so the line becomes softer. Sweep a bitter chocolate or charcoal-grey eye shadow into the crease of the eyelid, making sure that it does not extend above the crease line, and blend in well. Apply a natural-coloured eye shadow above the crease to the eye-brow or, for a more striking effect, use cooler colours, such as white, tones of grey and black, as they provide a stronger contrast to skin tone. Older skins, however, usually look better with softer, subtle eyeshades smudged into a smoky effect. Once your shadow is in place curl your lashes (see page 55) and apply two coats of mascara. For the evening you can afford to add a little touch of mascara to the outer edges of the lower lashes, which opens up the eyes and creates a frame for them, but don't overdo it and make the lashes look too heavy.

An age-old problem many of us encounter during a date is how to keep lipstick looking good through three courses and a bottle of wine. To make lipstick last all evening use a dark, neutral lip liner to both define and fill-in your lips. Carefully apply two coats of your chosen lipstick with a lip brush, blotting with a tissue between coats. Finish with a dab of shimmer or lip-gloss in the middle of the bottom lip for added allure. Lips are the obvious place to play up the glamour for evening, the perfect choices being shades of rich red and deep burgundy.

Short nails are the most elegant look for the evening. Nail colour can provide instant glamour: try 100 per cent true red or, for a softer look, two tones removed from that. If you have red-based skin tones the blue-reds or brighter orange-reds are more flattering, where-as people with more blue in their skin should try more brownish-reds. Certainly you can never go wrong with a French manicure using a pale, opalescent shimmer.

Glamour make-up is best saved for evening. Have fun with your evening look and experiment with different products until you have a selection that you adore. The right blend of products, colours and techniques will make you feel fabulous, sensuous and irresistible, which can only make the evening even more perfect.

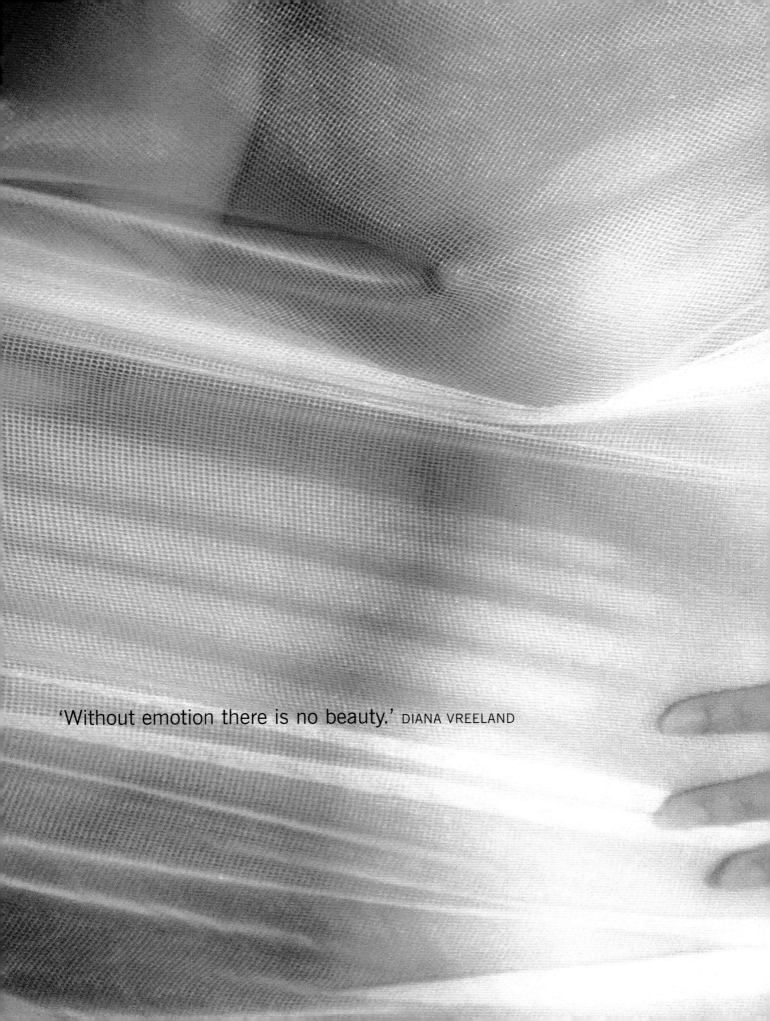

'Without emotion there is no beauty.' DIANA VREELAND

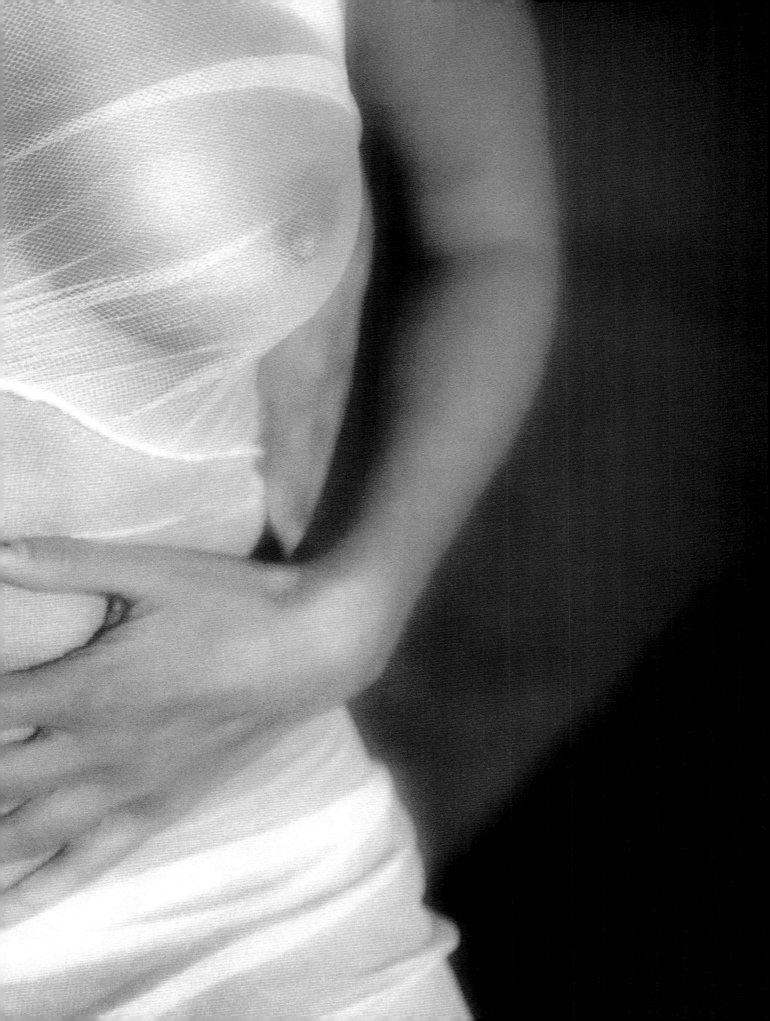

stillness

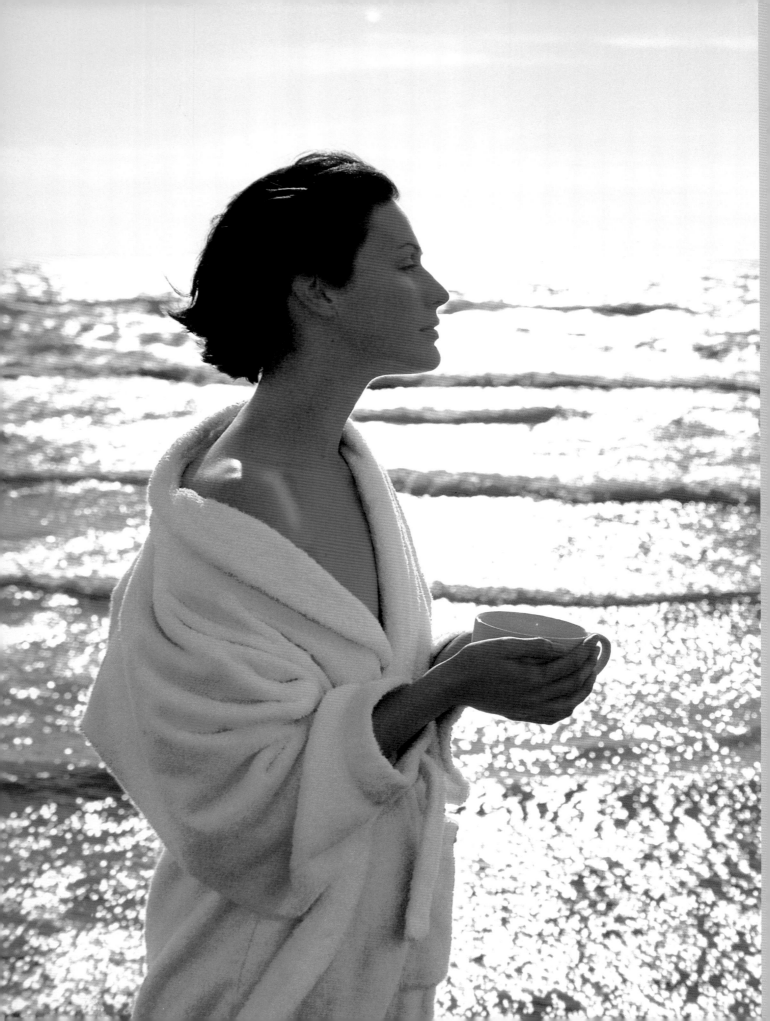

stillness

In the fast pace of the twenty-first century world, time seems to rush by, without us being able to catch our breath and enjoy the moment. We each need a place for peace and solitude, a place in which to dream, where time has no meaning and there is no commitment attached. Think of it as a decompression chamber, a place for meditation or for taking time out just to be. We should use this time and space to think of the day or focus our thoughts, to relax the body and stretch the mind.

Create a haven for yourself where you can be calm and quiet. Decorate your space with objects that you love or those that offer subtle sensory stimulation to make this your special place: create a comfort zone with calming colours; delight yourself with the delicate aromas of fragrant candles or exotic incense; soothe yourself with a cashmere throw or downy pillows, add a tiny altar or a picture of a person or place that has spiritual meaning for you. Adopt the Asian tradition of leaving your shoes, and the concerns of the outside world, at the front door of your retreat. Regular quiet time will free your mind, heal your body and make you able to deal more easily with stress and tension.

We spend a third of our lives in bed and for good reason: we need sleep in order to function properly when we are awake. When our regular sleeping pattern is disturbed it adversely affects our body, mind and spirit, resulting in our becoming more tense and stressed and therefore less able to sleep. With long working hours and a culture of constant entertainment we can often fall into the trap of believing that sleep is the least important part of our day. It is not surprising that stress and depression have become such wide-spread problems in our society. Entice yourself into sleep at night by sipping a soothing tisane made with calming and relaxing herbs, by taking a warm, aromatic bath or by placing lavender around your bedroom. When we are sick we sleep; when we are hurt we sleep; babies, teenagers and pregnant women sleep prodigiously. Sleep is our time for healing and growth; listen to your body and allow yourself to slumber.

Bathing has become a contemporary pastime. Use your time in the bath to still your mind and relax your body. When it comes to the evening wind-down, the Japanese take their bathing rituals very seriously. Bathing in Japan is a time to be alone and contemplative, to attain a state of mind and a reconnection with nature; it is about sensuality, wholesomeness and joy. Even the anticipation of a wonderfully relaxing, meditative soak in fragrant hot water can begin to release the tensions of the day. Cleanse, exfoliate, steam and envelop yourself in the aromas. Focus on the sounds of nature floating up through your window. Close your eyes; breathe; be calm.

home haven

A spiritually nurturing, calming environment should be free from clutter and the chaos of the outside world: you need a clear space for a clear mind. Colour can be used as an emotional tonic, whilst the juxtaposition of hard and soft, light and shade, rough and smooth can create a peaceful atmosphere.

Colour can be used to help infuse a room with the right mood, from soothing and cleansing white, pale blues or lilac tones to shades of violet, which pertain to spirituality, self-respect and dignity. Blue symbolises inspiration, devotion, peace and tranquillity, which makes it perfect to use to promote meditation and healing. It is also a cooling colour, creating a sense of space and slowing things down. Violet is an inspirational colour and can be helpful in attaining a higher state of consciousness.

Carpets and rugs offer a sense of emotional warmth that can be cosseting and nurturing; use fabrics and textures that are wonderful to walk on in bare feet, so you can feel softness on your soles. You may meditate while sitting on the floor, so rugs will ensure you feel safe and comfortable; perhaps place large cushions around you for support or snugness. Floor coverings also act as sound absorbers, muffling noise that could be distracting as you try to meditate or sit in peace.

Sound connects us to the world. What we mean by silence is the absence of intrusive sound, which is to some extent subjective. Generally speaking we are at peace when the sounds we hear are those that we want to hear or those that make us happy: use sound in your space to inspire you or focus your mind. Everybody has their own favourite music that touches the heart and warms the soul, but there are also sounds from nature, like the sound of the sea, which connect with some primitive yearning in most of us. Another sound that has an almost universal appeal, particularly when we are tucked up cosily inside our home, is that of driving rain against a skylight on a blustery evening, with the wind whistling through the trees.

Providing a focus to help still the mind and attune it to specific states of consciousness, music has proven to be a wonderful aid to meditation. Recent studies suggest that instrumental music, particularly when there is a constant tempo of 60 beats per minute, induces the relaxation response and can be an invaluable aid in reprogramming the subconscious with positive suggestions to aid healing and achieve personal goals. Experiment for yourself with some of the slow movements from Johann Sebastian Bach, such as *Largo* from the solo harpsichord concerto in C major or *Largo* from the concerto in G minor for flute and strings.

stillness

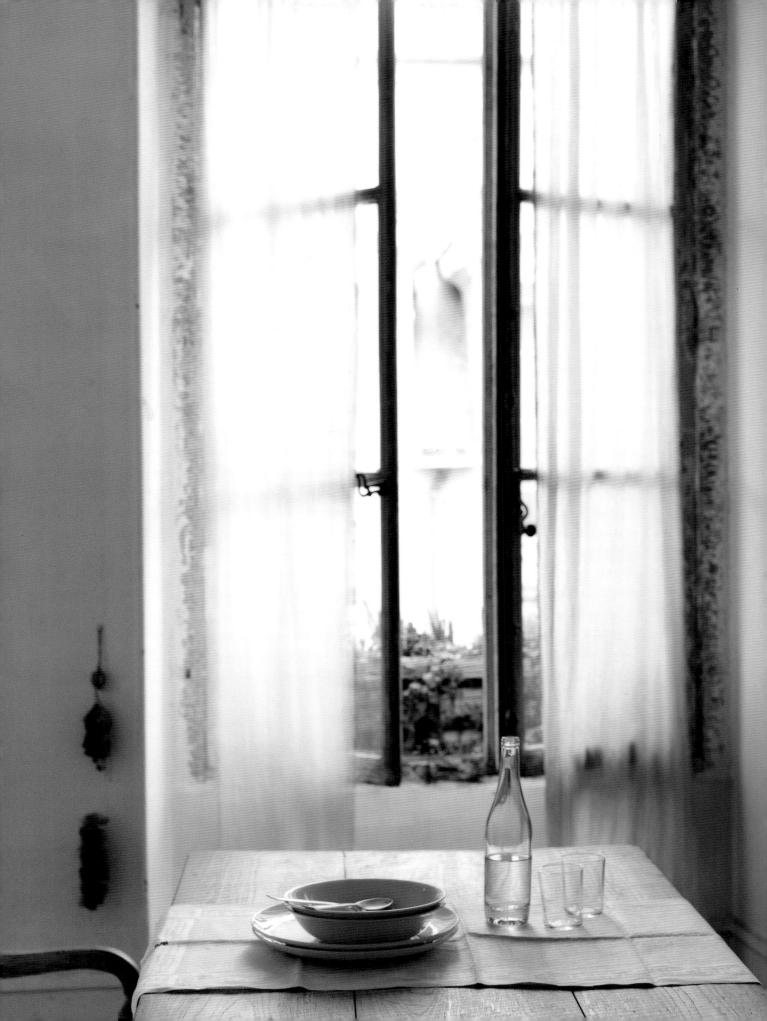

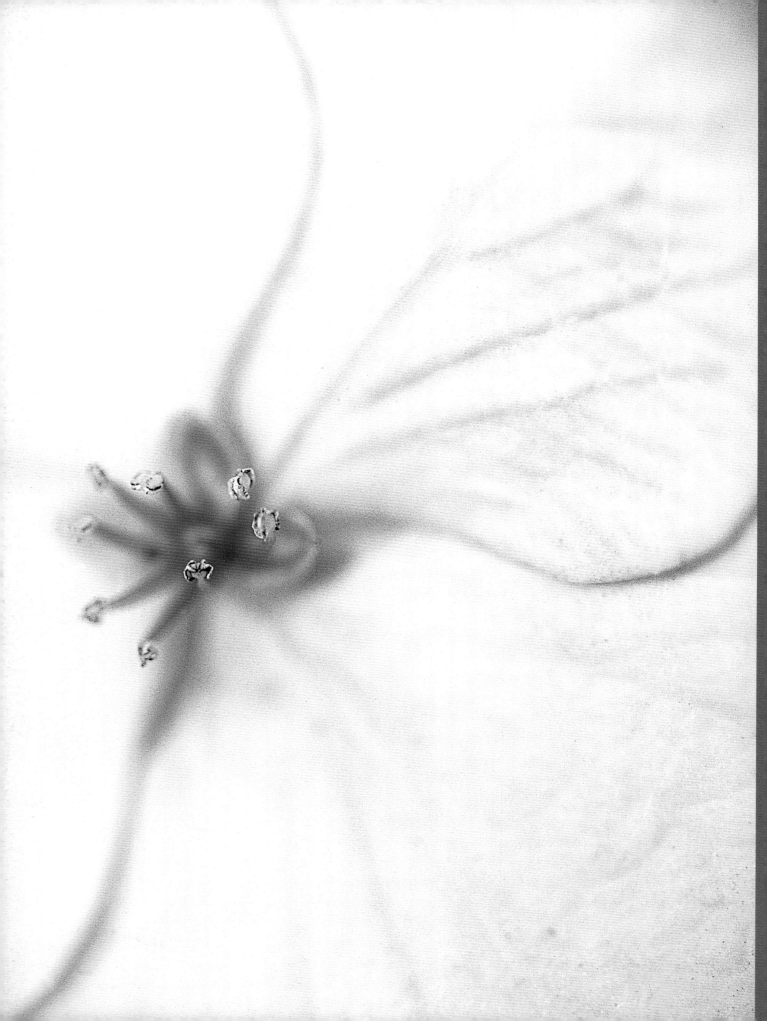

calming meditation

Throughout our history people of all religions and cultures have practised meditation to bring balance to their lives and promote personal growth. Meditation allows each of us to withdraw temporarily from the onslaught of daily pressures, tune in to an inner oasis of calm and create stillness in the mind. A few minutes of meditation each day can drastically improve our ability to cope with everyday life and help us to develop an awareness of our inner self. Anxiety and stress levels can be reduced effectively, concentration and rationality improved. Meditation also has a remarkable healing effect on the physical body and reduces high blood pressure. Even on a superficial level the benefits are obvious: when you are calm and relaxed you look better as you have no furrowed brows or frown lines.

Meditation involves a subtle act of 'letting go'. Like sleep, you are unaware you are meditating at the time; only recognising a meditative state once you have left it. During meditation the mind and its subject of concentration become one or samadhi – it is absolute. Regular practice calms the mind, relaxes the body and uplifts the soul.

There are two types of meditation: the first, which is usually the easiest, involves an external focus – most often an object, image, sound or symbol – which is used as a tool for concentration; the second type is abstract or formless meditation, which uses no external focus and consists of absorption in the self.

Practise meditation in your quiet, personal space where you will be warm, peaceful and undisturbed. Make a habit of meditating in this place so you learn to associate it with a state of focused concentration. Find a comfortable sitting position that can be held with minimal effort. You must be able to stay in your chosen position for a prolonged period without discomfort or it will be difficult for you to concentrate. The spine should be long, upright and balanced to allow energy to flow freely and to ease the awakening of the higher energy centres in the body. The classic posture for meditation is the full lotus, which keeps the body perfectly balanced. The legs are crossed and the feet rest on top of the opposite thigh with soles facing the ceiling. The legs and hips root down towards the earth and the spine rises effortlessly from this solid base. If you cannot do the full lotus try a half-lotus, which also has a pleasantly grounding effect but is a little uneven. For this reason alternate the lifted leg at each meditation session.

If you find it uncomfortable to sit on the floor for long periods begin by using a hard chair with a firm seat. Sit towards the edge of the chair with your back lengthened and your feet flat on the floor placed a little way apart. Rest your hands on your knees. You should feel balanced and at ease.

Hero pose is an ideal intermediate stage between sitting in a chair and sitting on the floor in one of the crossed-leg poses. The full posture requires considerable hip, knee and ankle flexibility but the following variation is suitable for most people. Kneel back on a pile of yoga blocks placed between your ankles. Use as many blocks as you need to feel comfortable, making sure that your sitting bones are perched just on the edge of them so that the thighs remain free. Keep your knees close together, your thighs parallel and the soles of your feet facing upward. Your head should now float weightlessly above your neck and it should be almost an effort to slouch.

stillness

Hand positions are a matter of personal choice. While sitting on a chair or in hero pose it is easiest to place your hands on your thighs with the palms facing down. You can also use your hands to make various seals, or mudra in Sanskrit, which seal energy into the body or conduct its flow in a certain direction rather like completing an electrical circuit. The classic mudra for meditation is known as the chin mudra or 'seal of consciousness'. Holding your index finger and thumb together with your palm upward to concentrate the flow of prana, the essential life force, toward the higher chakras or centres of spiritual power in the body aids concentration on the mind and the self.

Once you are in position begin your chosen meditation exercise. If you lose concentration guide your mind gently and uncritically back to the focus of the meditation, whether it is your breath, the flame of a candle or your mantra. Do not rush – the meditative state comes in its own time, so be patient and practice often. Start by aiming to meditate for 15 minutes a day and once you are able to do this gradually increase the length of the session to 30 minutes.

The biggest challenge is training the mind to achieve and maintain a single point of focus. A 'tool', such as your breath, a mantra or even something as simple as the flame of a candle, can help to concentrate the mind for successful meditation. At first you may find that you are simply concentrating on your chosen object, but with practice concentration turns into contemplation and eventually you and your object become indistinguishable and you experience the goal of meditation – perfect, unified stillness.

The following techniques engage your sense of hearing or sight to focus your mind. With experience it may be sufficient simply to imagine the sound or object.

breath-counting meditation
The breath is used to focus the mind. The sound of the breath forms its own natural mantra which is expressed as 'So-Hum' – the in-breath is said to make the sound 'So' and the out-breath 'Hum'. This is translated as 'I am' or 'I recognise my connection to my individual self and the greater, collective self, and the divinity within everything'. Meditation is a constant, gentle reminder of the connection between the individual self and the universal consciousness.

Close your eyes and listen to your breathing. Make no attempt to change its natural flow, just observe the breath as it is. Notice the point at which your breath touches the insides of your nostrils as you inhale and exhale. Begin to count your breaths from one to ten and back again using this counting routine as a way to keep your mind focused. After a time you can stop counting and just listen to the steady, rhythmic flow of your breath, which may become very slow during meditation. When your mind wanders bring it back to the breath. Resume counting if it helps you to concentrate.

meditation is a constant, gentle reminder of the connection between the individual self and the universal consciousness

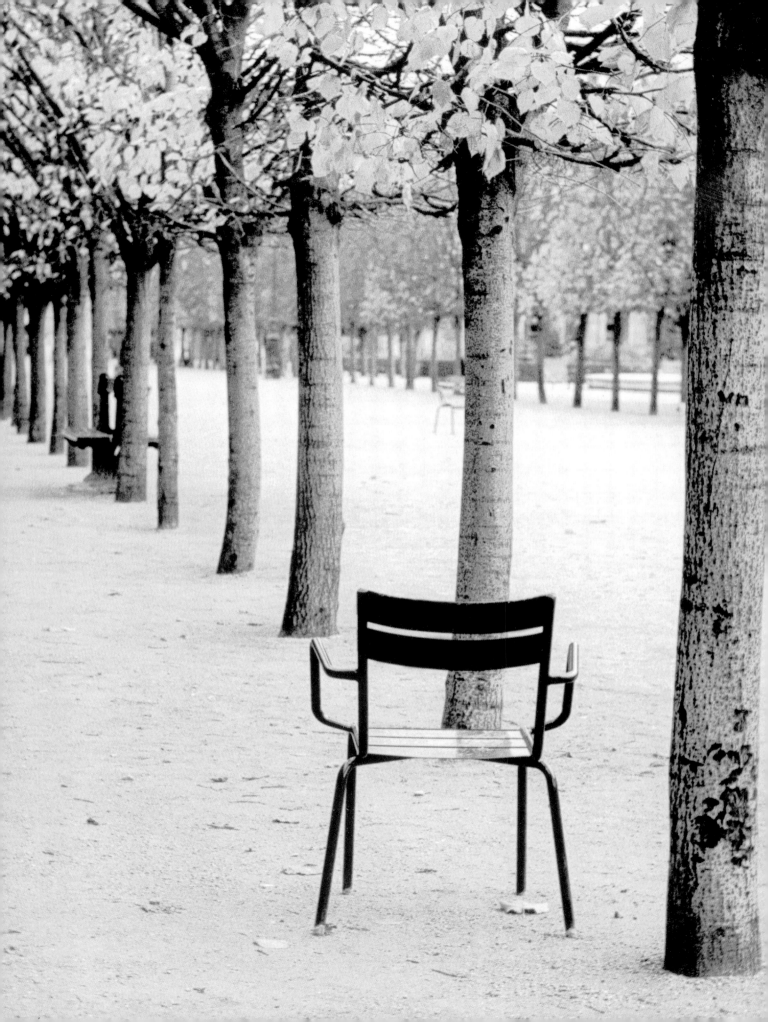

stillness

mantra meditation

Mantras are repeated words that help focus the mind during meditation. The word mantra means 'thought expressed as sound' and can be a single syllable, such as the holy syllable 'OM', or a set of words, phrases or sounds. Repeated aloud, the sound of 'OM' is said to be the nearest the human voice can come to the sound of the universal vibration.

There are different ways of using mantras, the most powerful being silent mental repetition, although they can also be whispered, spoken or chanted. In each case the purpose is to anchor the mind and experience the vibration of the mantra both physically and spiritually. Traditionally, your guru would give you a mantra and you should neither change nor disclose it to anyone. In the absence of a guru you can select your own mantra and repeat it to yourself during meditation or at any time to help calm and focus your mind. There are four things to consider when choosing a mantra: the sound of the words, the meaning, the idea that it embodies and its spiritual significance. Words such as 'love', 'peace' and 'harmony' are suitable mantras.

trataka

This is an exercise in concentration that leads you naturally into a meditative state. It is also a kriya or 'cleansing treatment' for the eyes. Please avoid this if you are epileptic.

Assume your meditation position and choose a static point or object to focus on. This should be roughly at eye level and can be an object such as a small statue. It can be wonderful to practise trataka outdoors in a natural environment, where you can choose a beautiful tree, or flower or mountain peak to focus upon. Gaze at your chosen object, keeping your eyes relaxed and steady. Do not stare or lose your point of focus – you are aiming to look clearly without strain. Keep gazing without blinking until your eyes start to water. When this happens, close your eyes and spend a few moments visualising your object behind closed lids on your forehead between your eyes. Open your eyes again and resume gazing at your object. Repeat this opening and closing of the eyes for several minutes. This level of concentration is excellent preparation for meditation; when you are experienced at it you can move seamlessly from concentrating on an object to being absorbed by it, which means you have reached a meditative state.

candle meditation

A candle flame is pleasant to focus upon and has symbolic qualities associated with light and ritual.

Sit in your chosen position and breathe naturally. Focus on a lighted candle and soften your gaze so that you are looking slightly beyond the flame. When you feel that you can retain the image of the candle flame in your mind's eye close your eyes and visualise it on your forehead between your eyes. At first the candle will fade and you will be left with nothing, so open your eyes and repeat the process. Eventually you will be able to retain the mental image for some minutes. When you achieve this level of concentration let go and lose yourself in the flame, enjoy the sense of spaciousness and expansion.

When you feel ready, open your eyes and come back to waking consciousness. Do not worry if you cannot keep the mind still – this comes readily with regular practise and you will find you have been meditating without realising it. Once you have achieved the meditative state you will immediately feel the benefits to your body and mind and in time discover a wonderful serenity and strength permeating your everyday life.

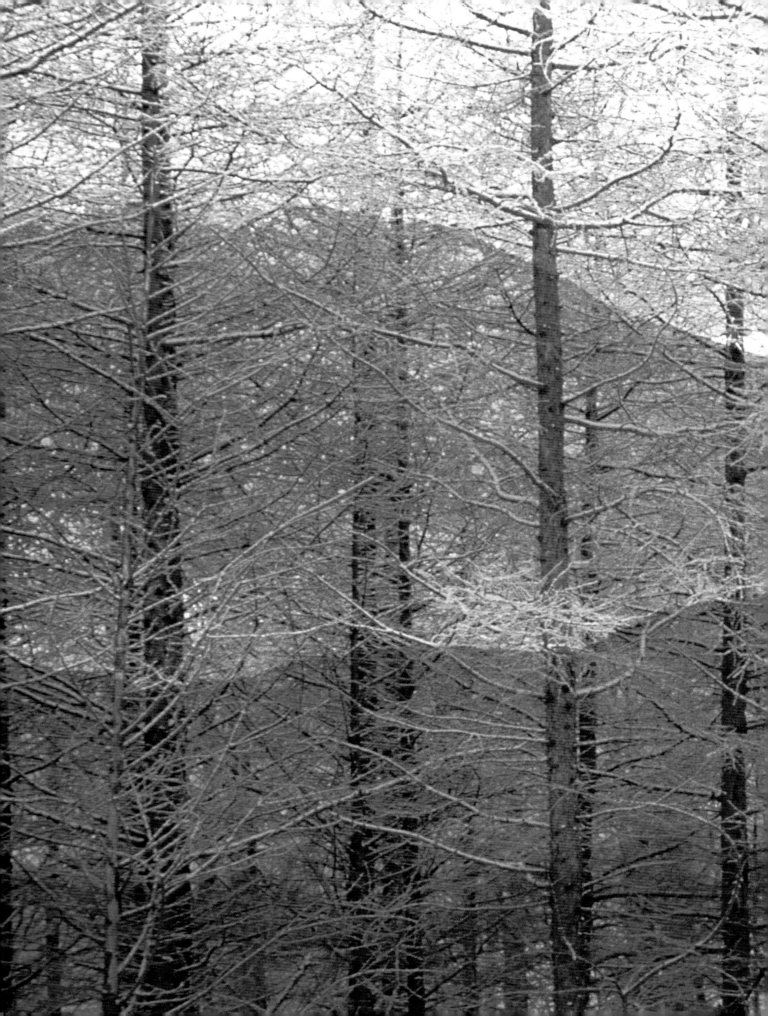

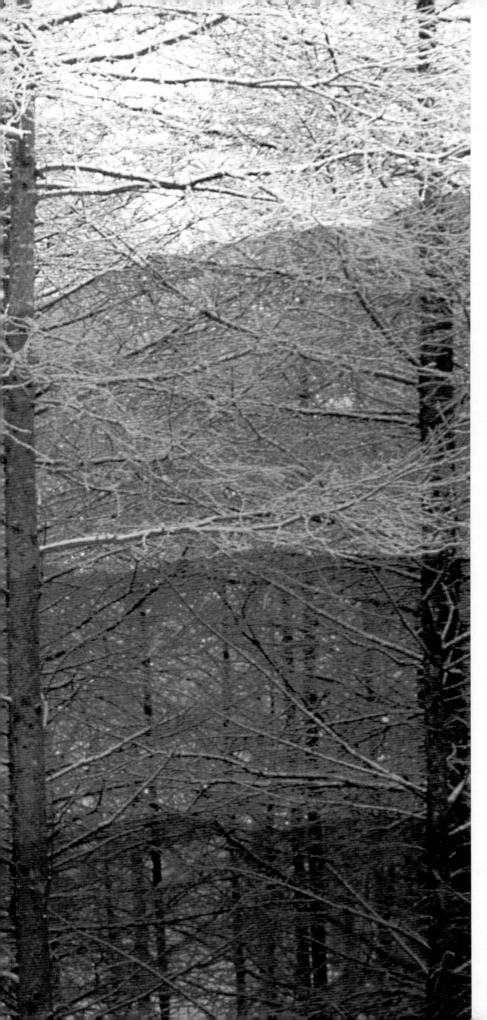

stillness

'no thought, no form,

only emptiness...

the joy of silence.'

ANON

bathing rituals

Too often in the West a bath is simply viewed as a place to cleanse the body, in Japan it is where one goes to cleanse the soul. Twenty-first century bathrooms are for physical, mental and emotional renewal and should be enticing. Hide away visually unappealing clutter in cupboards and create space for flowers, plants and natural objects. Peace lilies, daisies, bamboo and orchids are all efficient at expelling toxins and bring positive energy into the room. Stones, driftwood and organic shapes remind us of our intrinsic bond with the world outside our walls.

Each of the senses is engaged when bathing, and each glorious element should be well considered. Dimmer switches should be installed as a matter of course to allow flexibility in lighting levels – for an evening bath flickering, fragrant candlelight creates a warm, tranquil bathroom that is at one with the natural world.

Sounds, like scents, have the power to evoke moods and memories. Aiding relaxation, sound has the ability to transport us to a different world, if even for a moment in time. In Japan wind chimes are hung under the eaves to be stirred by the softest breezes; hang chimes outside your bathroom window to soothe and relax you while you bathe. Tranquil, natural sounds are the perfect complement to contemplative time spent in the bath, from a babbling brook or a soft waterfall to the gentle lap of waves on the shore. They create a fleeting moment of perfection – perfect because it is so fleeting. Experience for yourself the effects of playing music in the bathroom: music can be used as a soothing aural balm. Try gently uplifting Mozart, Thomas Otten's sensuous *Close to Silence* or the hauntingly beautiful *Dreamcatcher* by Secret Garden.

Touch is dependent on texture, temperature and the use of materials within the bathing space: ignite the senses with tactile surfaces. A warm stone floor underfoot; a soft headrest at the end of the tub; thick, Egyptian-cotton towels waiting on a heated towel rail. Feel the sensation on your skin when you apply your after-bath cream and choose clothes that enhance this feeling of silkiness and vitality.

use the scents of jasmine and rose to fragrance your bath and imagine that you are floating away in a tropical paradise

Smell is linked to the emotions and aromatherapy promotes a profound sense of wellbeing. In warm climates jasmine and roses are planted near bathroom windows to perfume the air: use these scents to fragrance your bath and imagine that you are floating away in a tropical paradise. The Romans were great advocates of aromatic bathing. Make your own herbal infusion by hanging a muslin bag filled with fresh or dry herbs under the hot tap as you fill the bath. Lavender, chamomile flowers, marjoram and rose petals all make wonderfully fragrant infusions. If you suffer from dry skin add some oat flakes or oat bran to the mix for an extra moisturising and softening effect. Essential oils can also be added to enhance the fragrance and calm or revive mind, body and spirit. After relaxing in a scented bath the body feels smooth and soft; the muscles and nerves begin to unwind from the tensions of the day.

relaxing evening bath Bathing promotes relaxation and induces restful slumber. Bathing in lukewarm water lowers the level of physiological tension and physical stimulation and helps shut down the entire body system. When you need to regroup after a long day and prepare for sleep try this relaxing bathing routine.

TO PREPARE AND USE THE BATH

Light a few lavender candles and place them around the bathroom, dim the lights and play Pachbel's *Canon in D major* softly in the background. To a warm bath add the following customised oil blend:

30ml sweet almond oil
3 drops geranium essential oil
3 drops lemon essential oil
4 drops sandalwood essential oil

Stir the water to ensure even dispersion of the oils before stepping in.

Lie back and relax in the bath water. Practise abdominal breathing for twenty minutes (see page 119), topping up the hot water as the bath cools.

Get out of the tub carefully, as it could be slippery underfoot, and dry the skin gently. Mix 20ml jojoba oil with 2 drops each lavender and sandalwood essential oils and massage into the skin.

Wrap up in a fluffy robe and relax for ten minutes before heading off to bed for an undisturbed night's sleep.

sleep solutions We all take sleep for granted but lack of sleep can cause depression, difficulty in weight regulation and over-production of stress hormones. Our need for an adequate amount of sleep is as non-negotiable as our need for exercise; for most people this means eight hours of sleep per night.

Sleeping is emphatically not a waste of time. During the first part of the night the complex chemical balances and controls within the body are restored. Then comes the Rapid Eye Movement or Dream State when the brain sifts through the day's experiences, enforcing memories and consolidating learning. The last period of sleep is crucial for creativity and mood; it is this part that depression deprives us of. Sleeping nourishes and renews body, mind and spirit.

Ease your body and mind into slumber with a relaxing evening bath scented with essential oils or by making your own flotation tank. Add 500g of Epsom's Salts, 250g of sea salt and one dessertspoon of clear iodine to your bath water. Lie back and relax for 20 minutes to feel the profound benefits of these healing salty waters. However, if you have recently shaved or have any open wounds, avoid this flotation bath until the broken skin has healed over.

Make sure you get some sunlight every day to reinforce the body's day–night cycle. Give yourself time to wind down before bed: don't exercise late in the evening as it can be stimulating; give your body time to expel caffeine by not ingesting it after lunch; eat dinner early so digestion is almost over by bedtime; and limit your alcohol consumption as it can dehydrate the body and cause wakefulness. Before bed, drink a glass of warm milk with a little sugar and a pinch of ground turmeric: milk activates sleep-inducing chemicals in the brain and acts as a natural tranquilliser; turmeric has antiseptic properties that calm throat irritations and reduce phlegm that can keep you awake. Keep a notepad next to your bed so that if you find thoughts going round your head you can write them down and then forget them for the next 8 hours.

stillness

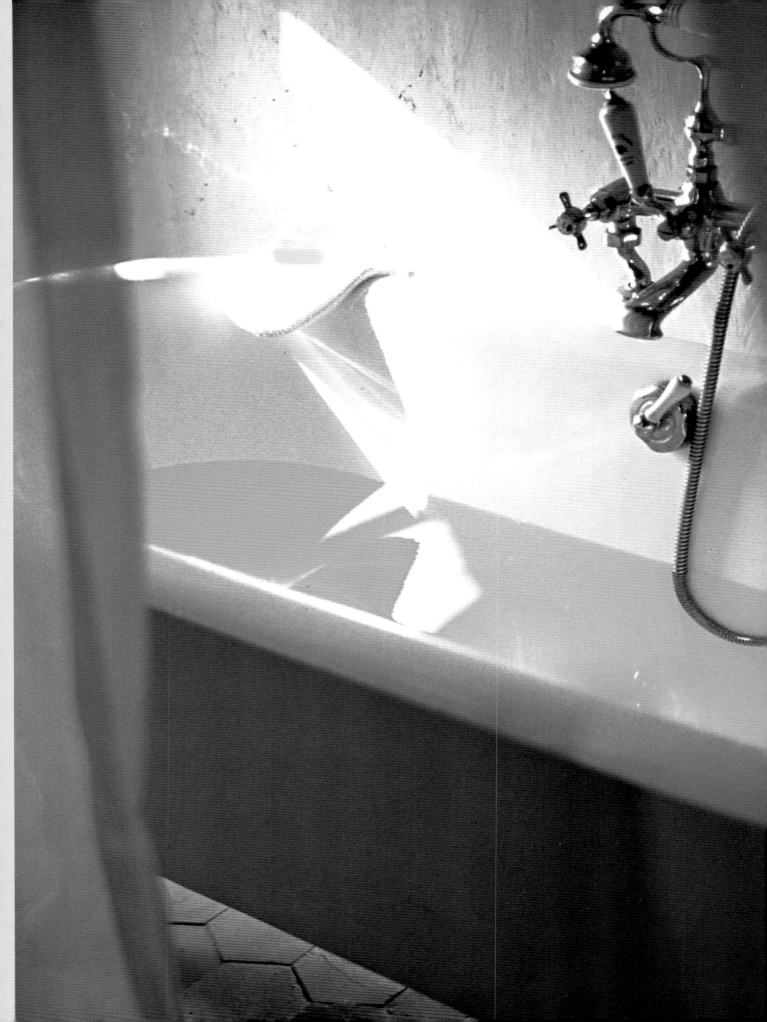

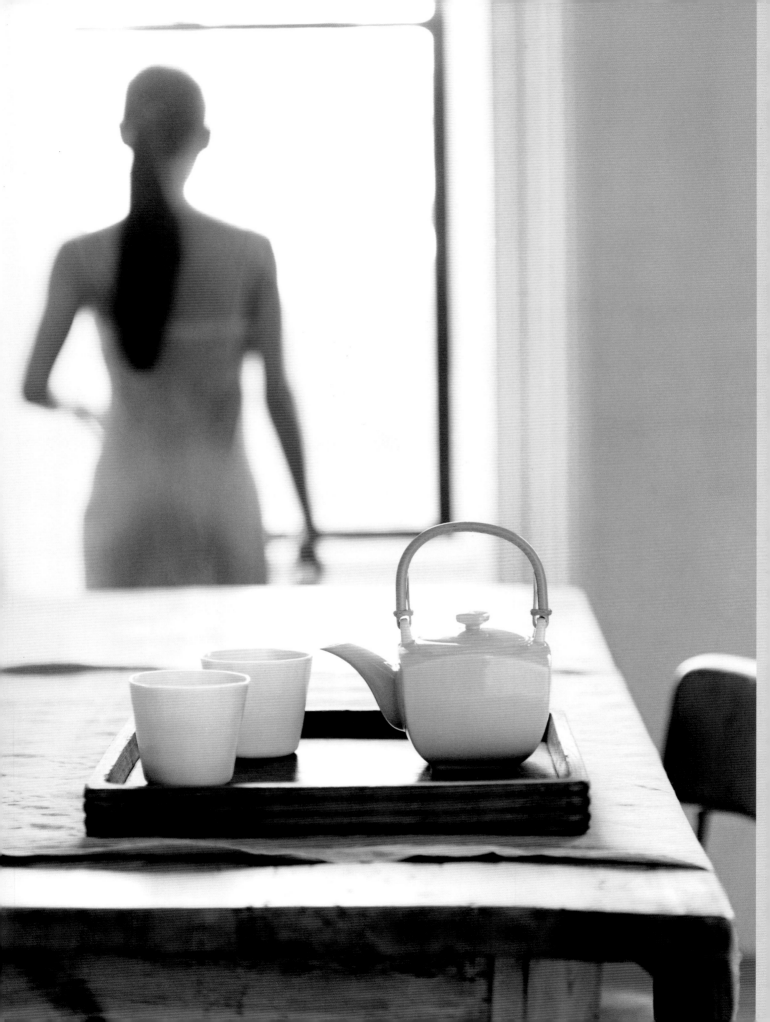

slumber-inducing tisane

Try the following herbal tisane for a mild sedative effect.

TO PREPARE THE TISANE

2 teaspoons dried chamomile flowers
2 teaspoons dried lavender flowers
2 teaspoons dried catnip leaves
2 cups boiled water

Place the herbs in a teapot and pour over the boiling water. Cover and steep for 10 minutes. Strain and sweeten with honey to taste.

Sip slowly while hot.

relaxation brew

Another delicious infusion to end the day.

TO PREPARE THE TISANE

2 teaspoons dried mint leaves
2 teaspoons dried chamomile flowers
2 teaspoons dried catnip leaves
2 teaspoons dried crushed hops
½ teaspoon cut dried valerian root
3 cups boiled water

Place the herbs in a teapot and pour over the boiling water. Cover and steep for 10 minutes. Strain and sweeten with honey to taste.

Sip slowly while hot.

relaxing tisanes

Insomnia is a plague of modern-day living. The pressure of the daytime battle against the clock can be difficult to lose at bedtime. Lifestyle changes will bring great improvement – after a day of physical exertion the body will crave its rest at bedtime. Nevertheless overexcitement, mental turbulence or excessive exhaustion can make falling asleep difficult.

Tisanes made from fresh or dried herbs are the perfect way for the mind and body to slow down before bedtime. Their delicate aromas and subtle flavours calm and soothe us, while their herbal properties gently ease us into sleep.

We slow down to measure the herbs; there is time for reflection while the kettle boils and the herbs steep. We can then sit cradling the warm cup in our hands, feeling the texture of the ceramic, inhaling the heady aromas. When the leaves, seeds, roots and fruits of herbs meet very hot water their volatile oils containing the aroma, taste and medicinal value of the plant are released. The very essence of each herb is transferred into the water to be sipped by us for sheer enjoyment or healing.

stillness

balance

balance

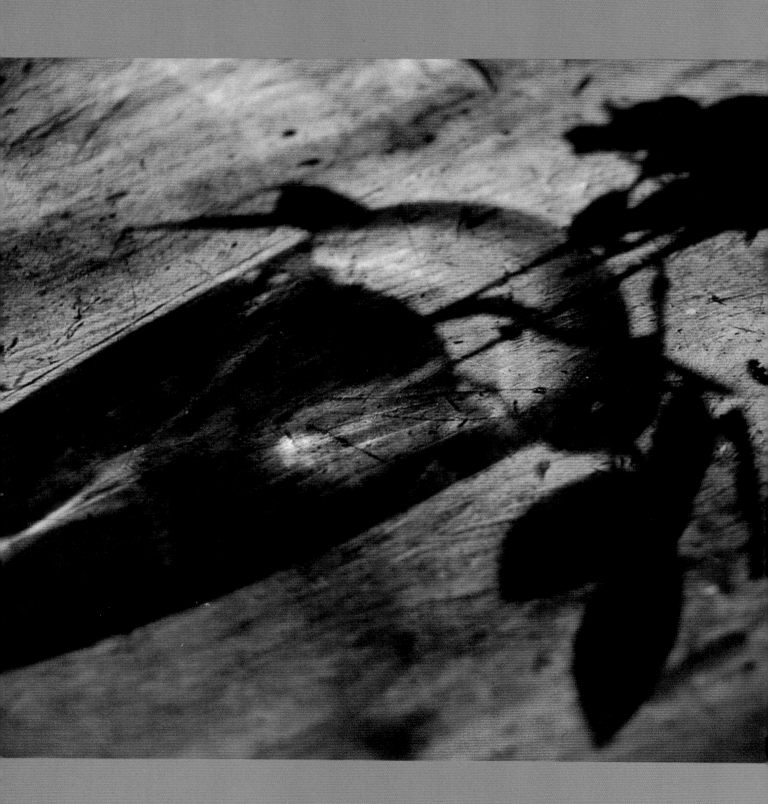

balance

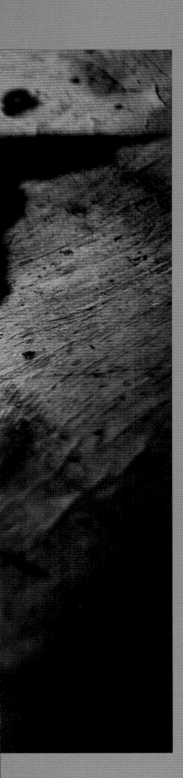

Stress is bound up in our preoccupation with doing more things in less time. Multi-tasking is wreaking havoc on our health; respecting our cultures and traditions, building a career, nurturing family and friends (let alone ourselves), experiencing the arts and enjoying nature all take time. It is essential that we take a step back from our hectic schedules once in a while to remind ourselves of what is important: to live well and healthily, to enjoy all that life has to offer, to feel free and be inspired. Living a balanced life cannot be rushed.

Balance can be achieved in every area of our lives, from the spaces that we inhabit to the food that we eat. The home is a sanctuary for contemplation and relaxation and should nurture both body and soul. Pared-down interiors following Zen or feng shui principles are simple and stress-free, with soothing natural textures providing comfort and sensory stimulation. Music has the power to bring peace and create harmony: resonant monastic chants and drums of distant cultures connect to something buried deeply within us, a universal equilibrium.

We need to find physical, mental and spiritual release from the daily rush if we are to be happy. Movement therapies such as yoga and t'ai chi, which take their lead from ancient eastern philosophies, promote physical strength, mental awareness and spiritual freedom. Bodywork techniques, such as an aromatherapy massage with hormone-rebalancing rose geranium essential oil, utilise the healing power of touch and scent to restore equilibrium and flood the body with vital energy. In this modern world we also need to rebalance ourselves internally: the detoxification process cleanses the system, boosts our energy and sharpens our senses of taste and smell so that we enjoy even more the fresh, vibrant flavours of the foods we love.

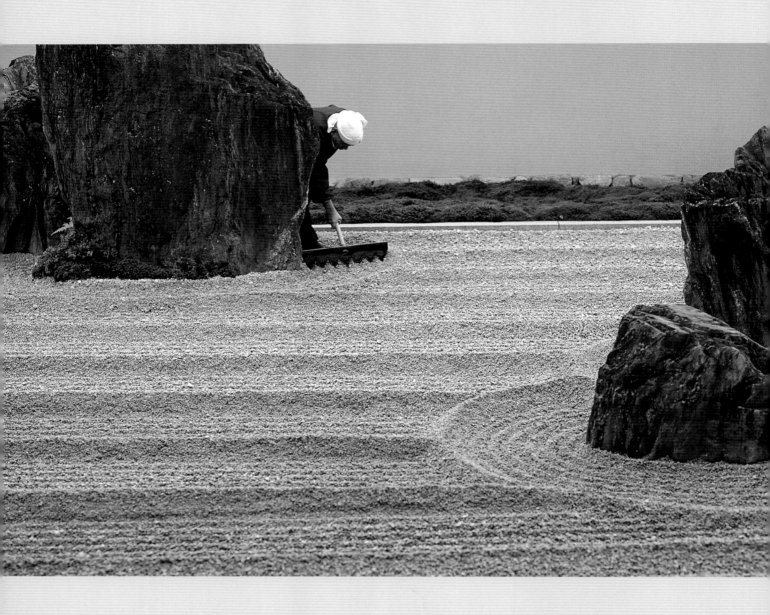

zen principles
The traditional Japanese understanding of beauty and worth is based on the simple things in life; it promotes honour and respect for the spirit and the power of nature. Zen is a way of life not a belief. It is pure, sentient awareness that allows us to look at life from a fresh perspective. Zen provides a road to self-discovery through a process of self-realisation; by exposing our self-imposed illusions we gain a better understanding of our true nature.

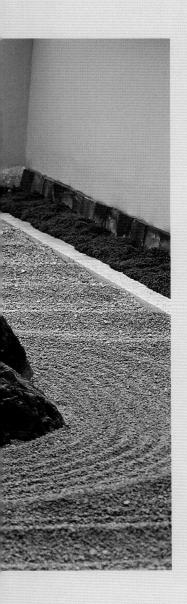

Zen teaches awareness, that we should pay full attention to the smallest details of life. It promotes mindfulness, so that we become aware of actions as well as their consequences. Zen encourages a sense of purpose by making sure we perform actions for their own sake with all our attention and commitment. We should not compare, disparage or discriminate, but learn to see beyond the form of the object to its very spirit. Zen brings lightness to life, a sense of calm, an eye for beauty. Spontaneity and freedom transform mundane events into the extraordinary. The trick is to transform menial tasks into life's rewarding rituals.

Consider the design and layout of the immediate surroundings of a building. Plants provide not only colour but also architectural shape and form. Residential gardens are now being restructured to complement the interiors of houses, extending living space outdoors. Gardens are spaces for contemplation, escape and refuge; they provide us with safety valves in today's high-pressure world.

In distant cultures elements of the natural world have great symbolic meaning. Raindrops are considered pearls of wisdom, which are there for all of us to learn from if only we take the time to look. The lotus plant is known as the 'ho', or harmony, flower in Chinese and is a metaphor for the mystery of life. It represents hope and inspiration, the spiritual awakening of the heart. It is a physical reminder of the strength that lies within to overcome the problems of life and achieve perfection. Bamboo is both beautiful and practical as it allows favourable chi energy to circulate. It symbolises fidelity, wisdom and longevity and, together with plum, orchid and chrysanthemum, comprises the Chinese 'four noble plants' that symbolise happiness. Harmony and balance are central to the Chinese notion of health and wellbeing. They embrace the Taoist concept of Yin and Yang, two opposing bodily forces animated by chi energy – the breath of life.

balance

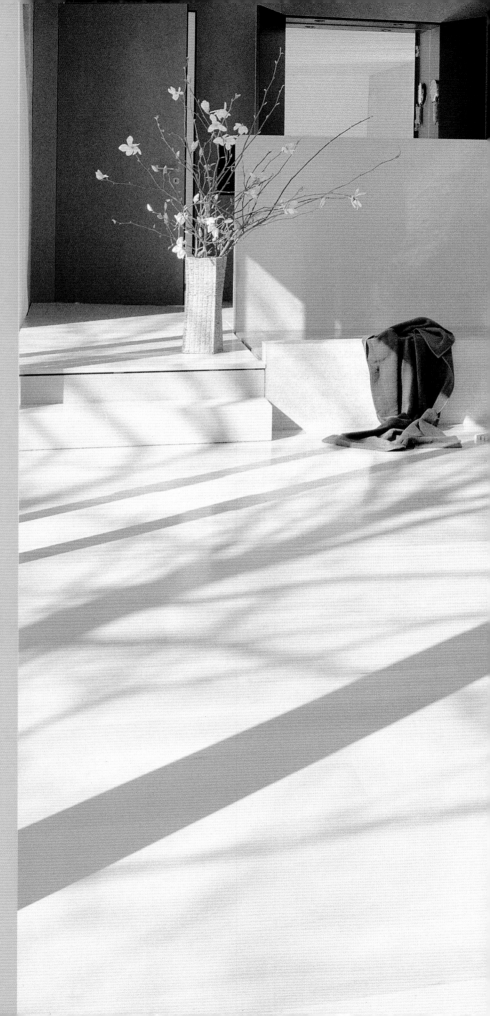

restful retreat

Home is our heartland, a place to restore the delicate balance between mind and body, where we can be ourselves without pretension.

We all need space for solitude, for contemplation, a place in which to relax, to meditate, to create or simply to dream. Your home is your own personal space in the world, so why not make it your inner sanctuary? Use the space and décor to stimulate the senses and provide an uninterrupted flow of energy through your home. Natural colours and textures are calming and soothing for the senses. Objects from the natural world exude positive energy that rebalances our body and mind. Music has the power to excite, inspire and uplift the soul; think of sonorous Tibetan chants, mystical Gamelan music from Bali and Native American drumbeats that touch the very animal core of our being.

balance

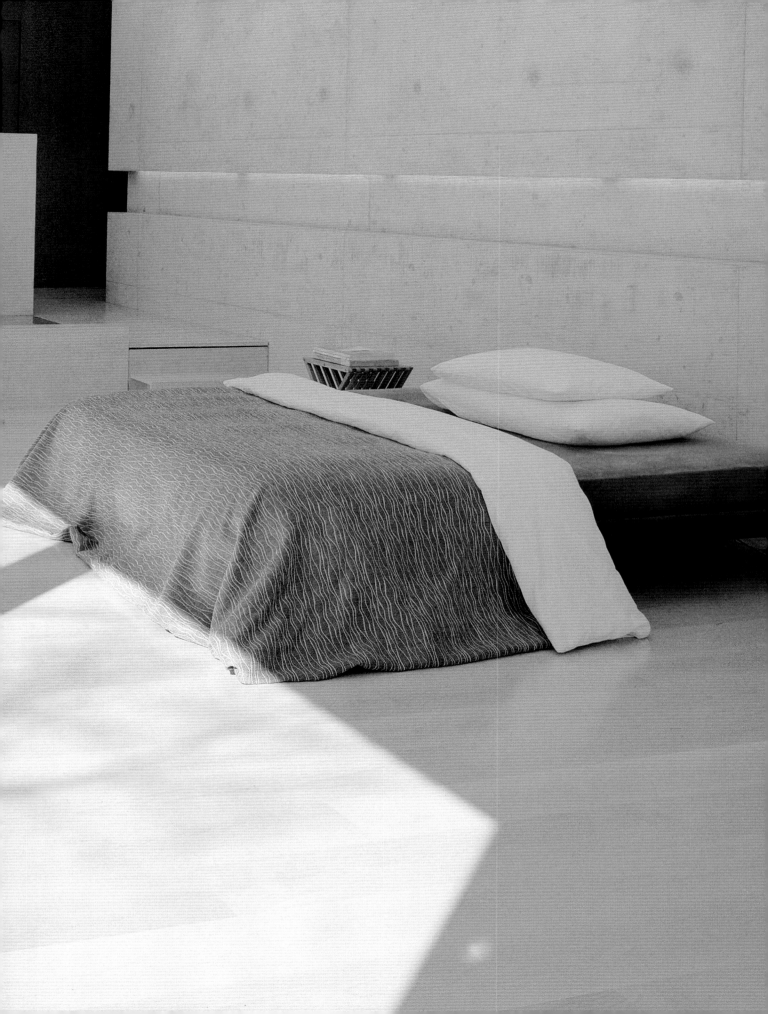

attention to detail

Simplicity in design fulfils our need to seek tranquillity and sanctuary from the rigors of an exacting and severe existence. We need to create space for spiritual reflection and fulfilment of inner needs. Ambient lighting brings harmony and positive energy. Gentle, natural fragrance relaxes and uplifts. A colour palette inspired by nature evokes serenity.

Surround yourself with objects that are meaningful to you and that appeal to all your senses: the tactile pleasure of soft cushions, the comforting embrace of a cashmere throw, the aromatic indulgence of essential oils or the intense, spiritual pleasure of incense. Colours carry an important resonance in our interiors and neutral earth tones – beige and taupe, through brown, grey and black – help to ground and rebalance us, offering a subliminal sense of protection. Firelight creates a happy and vital atmosphere acting as a tonic for the immune system. Yellow light warms and energises, removing emotional energy blocks and building self-confidence.

'Less is more' in the balanced interior, but what little there is must be perfect. Value beautiful, much-loved possessions and display them in a way that enhances their perfection. Space containing only the bare essentials also accentuates the sensuality of surfaces and finishes. This is best exemplified in the sublime harmony and balance in minimalist interiors, where the opposing sensations of textures and natural finishes provide pleasure and stimulation. Japanese 'wabi sabi' refers to an appreciation of simple, everyday items used in a refined manner. It induces a desire to revoke everything worldly in favour of the wonders of nature and mystical contemplation of life. Objects from nature, particularly flowers, can provide a source of wonder when brought into the home. Display the true beauty of each flower by using Ikebana, the minimalist Japanese art of flower arranging.

A simple, natural environment fosters a corresponding lifestyle. When everything is stored away a beautiful simplicity and sense of calm instils the atmosphere. Make changes in your home that will reverberate positively in your life. Perhaps one day, architects and designers will produce homes with spirit and soul, understanding the concept of chi energy and recognising the true impact of colours, textures and form. Until that day it is down to us to create environments that nurture our innermost needs.

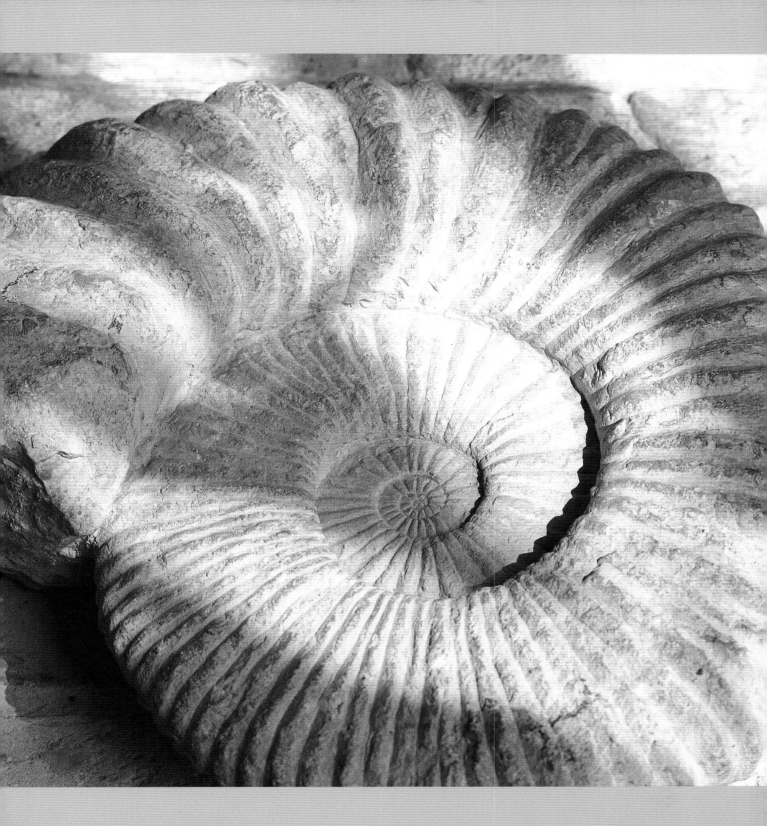

balance

harmonious interiors

Feng shui is our intuitive response to space. It ensures that the energy, or chi, that moves around our homes like an invisible breath is of a consistently high quality and is kept moving at a healthy pace. Deep within us we do know what best suits our personal needs, the best place to sit or eat, the design and colours that will help us to relax, the forms that keep us focused, but somehow this intuition has been lost in the mad-paced, man-made fabric of our society.

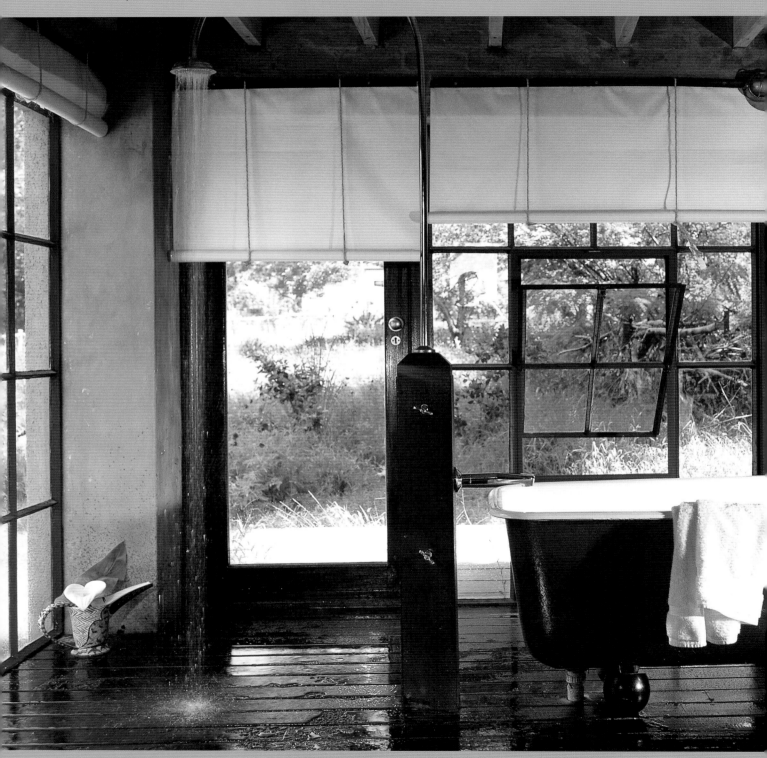

balance

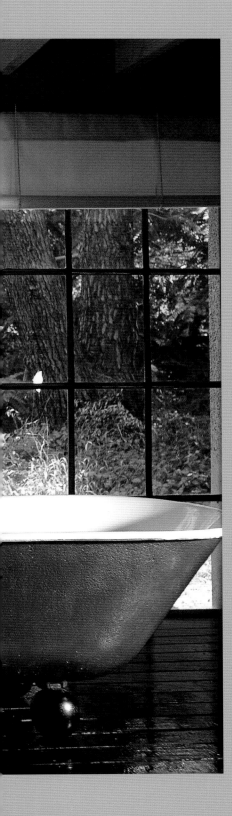

THE HALLWAY should be welcoming and bright. Leave shoes here to stop outdoor energy entering your inner sanctuary. Shiny door fittings encourage chi (energy) into the home.

THE LIVING ROOM should always have enough space for people to congregate comfortably. To avoid headaches do not place a seat directly under a ceiling beam. Hard, sharp edges on furniture can prevent relaxation, so avoid glass-topped tables. Make a fireplace, not the television, the focal point of the room and emphasise it by placing a mirror above.

THE KITCHEN should be a bright, open space with smooth lines and curves to encourage an even flow of chi. Use natural materials wherever possible; stainless steel kitchens can be stressful environments. The cooker, sink and refrigerator should form a triangle to maintain a balance between their different energies. Eat in a calm, comfortable space without clocks to create a timeless, unhurried dining environment. A round dining table draws people together and promotes conversational flow.

THE HOME OFFICE when kept orderly, is empowering, as an uncluttered environment promotes clarity of thought. Empty waste paper bins daily to avoid stagnation. Position a cleansing plant, such as a poinsettia, spider or jade plant, beside a computer to counteract debilitating electro-magnetic discharges. Use an ioniser to boost negative ions.

THE BATHROOM can be a negative space, so ensure that all the plumbing is in top condition and use tall, upright plants to counteract the energy that it drains away. Position a large mirror so that you can see as much of yourself as possible; a split reflection can affect health and add to indecision.

THE BEDROOM, if facing west, is preferable for people who find it difficult to settle, whilst rooms facing sunrise are ideal for those who have problems waking up. Position your bed with care, with a solid wall behind you rather than an open area or window. Give yourself a clear view of the door, using a mirror to do so if necessary. Avoid sleeping directly in line with the bedroom door, or you will be lying in the path of energy as it enters the room.

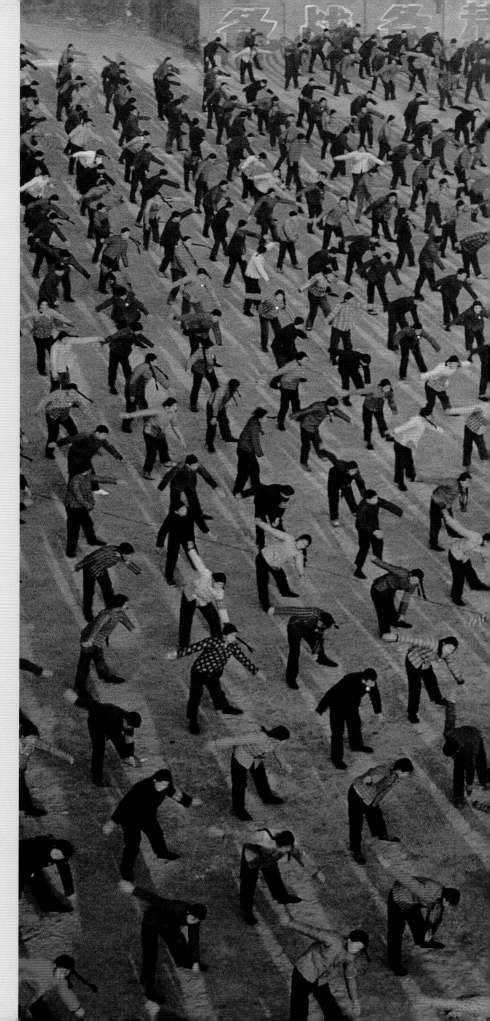

'We cannot change
the world,
but we can definitely
transform ourselves.
Self-transformation
is essential,
not the transformation
of the world.'

SWAMI RAMA

balance

114

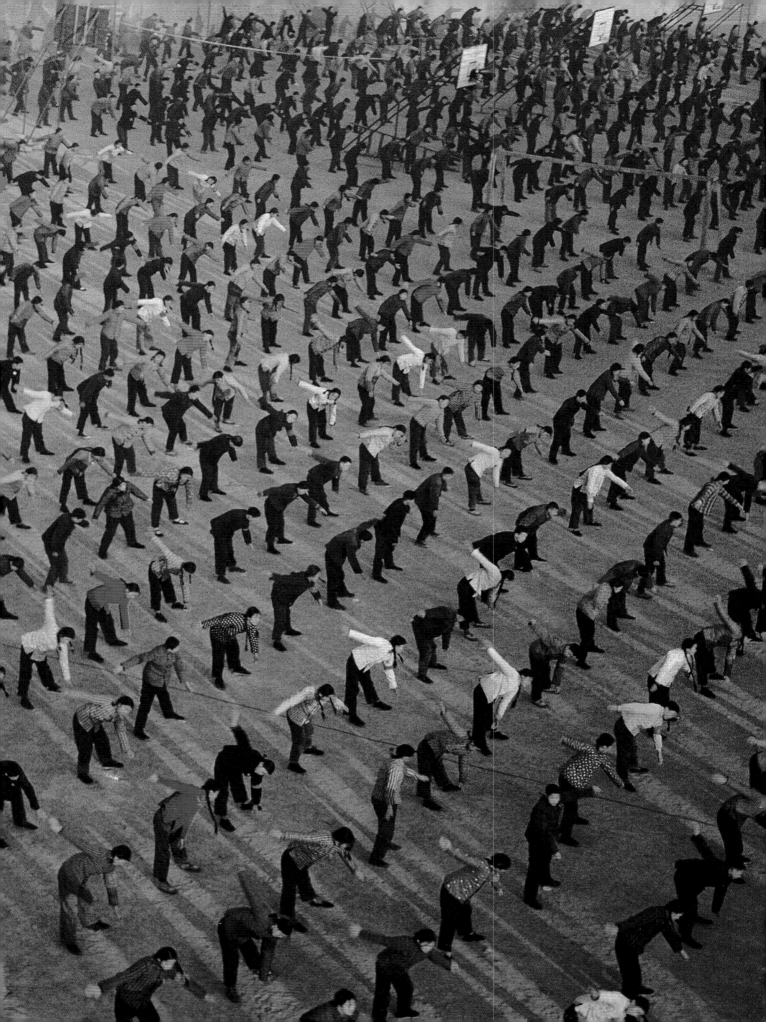

movement therapies

Regular exercise can bring both mental and physical change by relieving stress and rebalancing the body. For many people movement work is the most satisfying and intuitive path to fitness and stress relief. Movement therapies from t'ai chi to yoga focus inwardly on the restoration and cultivation of physical balance, stability and symmetry. Most therapies harmonise movement with breathing. Synchronising the two requires complete concentration, which calms and soothes the mind and enhances sensual awareness.

'The secret of life is balance,

and the absence of balance

is life's destruction.'

HAZRAT INAYAT KHAN

Movement therapy techniques improve strength, flexibility, co-ordination and balance and teach individuals to correct their own bodies. Quality of movement and postural alignment is determined over the years. When we are tense or sustain an injury, including psychological trauma, our muscles automatically contract in preparation for flight or defence. Sustained contraction leads to shortening of the muscles, constricted breathing and decreased blood-flow to the organs. To counteract this long-term tension all movement therapies follow the same basic paths:

BREATHING – one of the few autonomic systems that we can consciously override. When we breathe deeply we send nutrient-rich, oxygenated blood to heal and revitalise our tissues and a message to every system in the body that it can relax.

RELEASING – lubricates the joints and facilitates blood flow to the tissues with stretches, muscle-balancing and range-of-motion exercises.

CORE STRENGTH – firms back muscles and provides abdominal and pelvic-floor support to the lower back and pelvis. As alignment improves and the lower trunk muscles strengthen, overworked individual muscles unclench taking the strain off distorted joints and pressure off irritated nerves.

STRENGTH/ENDURANCE – helps maintain and increase bone density.

CARDIOVASCULAR – promotes heart health, lowers cholesterol, stabilises blood-sugar levels, improves circulation and burns fat at an increased rate.

MEDITATION AND VISUALISATION – reduces stress, increases self-understanding, improves awareness of the body's signals and leads to a greater sense of spiritual connection and wellbeing.

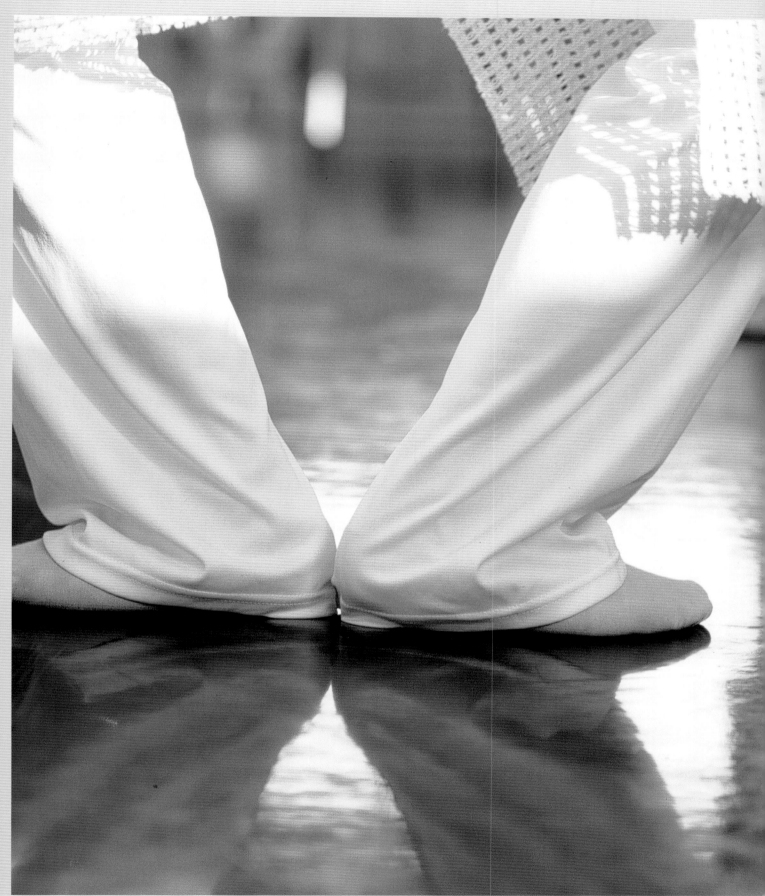

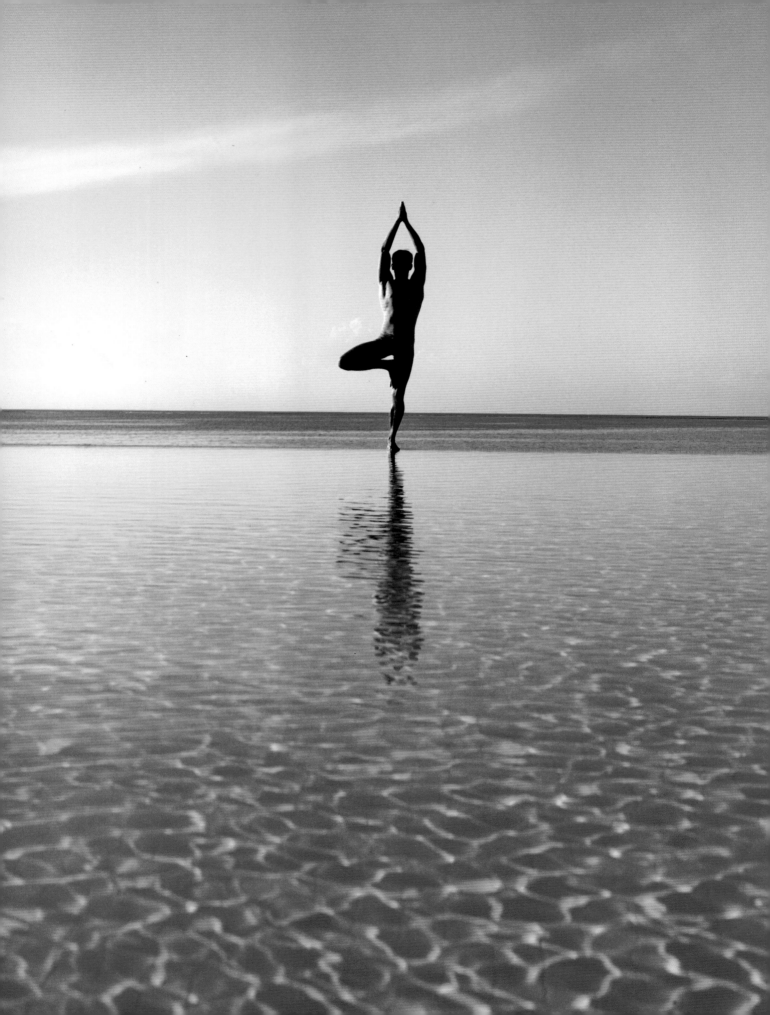

breath of life

By learning to observe and control our breathing we can influence our emotional state, our ability to concentrate and our energy. Breath control is an essential part of yoga practice: it is only by extending the breath that we can learn to channel prana and reach higher states of consciousness.

The basic function of breathing is to bring energy into the body, but most people do not breathe in a way that utilises all the space in their lungs. According to one yogic tradition the number of breaths in a lifetime is predetermined and so by slowing down the breath, life can be prolonged. This may seem far-fetched, but slowing down our breathing does reduce stress levels enabling us to relax and enjoy life more fully.

Moods and emotions are closely linked with breathing patterns: states of agitation cause the breath to be quick, shallow and uneven, which then exacerbates the original anxiety; when we feel relaxed we breathe more slowly and evenly. Pranayama, or energy control, is a breath-control technique that develops the ability to calm and control the breath to focus the mind and manage the emotions. It is known to have enormous curative value by increasing the intake of oxygen into the body and blood stream so that all the internal organs gain the nourishment they need. Practice strengthens breathing muscles, helps to expand lung capacity and frees the mind from the obstructions of negative or wandering thoughts.

pranayama is divided into three phases: inhalation, breath retention and exhalation. The inhalation is the nourishing breath that brings energy, warmth, strength and vitality to the mind and body. Breath retention creates a clear pathway around the body to be filled with energy. The exhalation is cleansing, cooling, restorative, calming and balancing. The first stage in pranayama is the non-judgemental observation of your natural breathing. Once you have gained a basic awareness of your breath, you can learn specific exercises that will develop the control you have over your body and mind.

kapalabhati is an exercise in diaphragmatic control that uses a 'pumping' breath action to produce mental clarity. The exercise strengthens the diaphragm, tones the heart, liver and stomach and clears out blockages so that energy and oxygen can flow freely. Kapalabhati, like most breathing exercises, should be practised in rounds.

Start by taking a couple of normal breaths. Inhale deeply through your nose. Now sharply contract your abdominal muscles to forcefully exhale through your nose, as if you were blowing out candles but through your nose. As your diaphragm releases you will automatically inhale gently. Repeat the pumping action of the exhalation together with the passive in-breaths in four short, rhythmic bursts. Then take a deep breath and exhale normally. This is one round of kapalabhati. Repeat this 4 more times gradually building up to 4 rounds of 20 breaths.

ujjayi breathing is a simple exercise used during postural practice, particularly in ashtanga vinyasa yoga. The technique consists of making a gentle, continuous hissing sound on both the in-breath and the out-breath by contracting your throat muscles slightly. The sound, similar to the sea, provides the focus for the breath. As the pressure of the breath is controlled it becomes very slow and even. Ujjayi has a tranquillising effect, renews energy and concentration, tones the respiratory system and internal organs and increases body heat. To practise making the sound, breathe out through your mouth making a soft 'haaa' noise, and then try to make the same noise with your mouth closed so that you are exhaling through your nose. Breathe in through your nose trying to replicate the sound. Repeat 12 breaths and gradually increase this. Ujjayi breathing should be audible but not necessarily loud.

brahmari focuses attention on exhalation and can be profoundly relaxing. Inhale fully through the nose. On exhalation make a rounded and steady humming sound. Listen to the hum and vary its pitch, moving the sound around inside your head and chest until it feels comfortable. Make this sound on each exhalation starting with 5 breaths and building up gradually.

chi gong, along with acupuncture, massage and herbal therapy, is one of the four pillars of Chinese Herbal Medicine. This slow, flowing meditation-in-motion focuses on mastery of the breath: 'chi' or 'qi' means breath of life or energy and 'gong' denotes cultivation or control. It is a gentle, calming discipline; with regular practise it promotes full integration of mind and spirit and can be very helpful in regulating emotions, inducing self-healing and maintaining wellness.

t'ai chi, developed from traditional forms of chi gong, translates as 'big energy'. The movements are soft and flowing, developing inner strength and energy. Synchronisation of breath and movement encourages balance and focus as well as an understanding of the movement of energy within the body and a sense of the body's relationship to the space around it. It is also a self-realisation discipline that encompasses all aspects of life, bringing balance and moderation.

alexander technique corrects the build-up of muscular tension that tends to develop into bad postural habits. Patterns of habitual movement can be changed

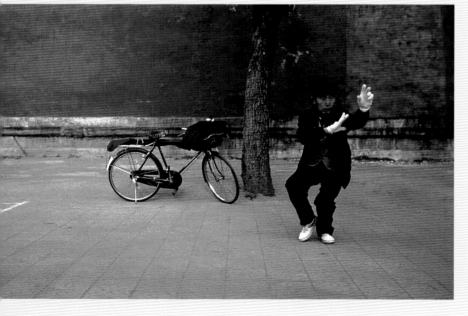

to release stress, improve alignment and body image, and eliminate pain and tension.

aqua therapies are pool-based movement and treatment therapies that can benefit those with joint or back pain. The compressive effect of immersion has a tonic effect on the whole body: it assists muscle blood flow, helps rid the muscles of metabolic waste and causes changes in the renal system that help lower blood pressure.

pilates leads to increased power, muscle integration and flexibility with special emphasis on the 'powerhouse' muscles of the abdomen, pelvic floor, lower back, inner thighs and buttocks. All the exercises are anatomically precise, leading to an understanding of the body as a whole; practitioners learn to identify and release all unnecessary tension when working specific muscle groups and joints. Muscle control determines the quality of each movement and is key to making progress as well as to avoiding injury. The totality of this action builds stamina without overloading any single group of muscles and builds a protective sheath for the vulnerable lower spine. By working through a carefully controlled series of graceful movements, improvements can be made to circulation, range of motion, co-ordination, flexibility, strength and posture.

yoga dates from 2800BC, making it the most ancient method of personal development. It encourages focus and the awareness of internally flowing energy. The six main paths of yoga approach the ultimate goal of self-realisation by a different route, but they are all based on the premise that human beings can, through their own actions, become one with the Absolute:

JUNANA YOGA – the path of wisdom; the main practices are study and meditation.

BHAKTI YOGA – the path of devotion; most suited to people who are attracted to prayer.

balance

KARMA YOGA – the path in which the practitioner devotes him or herself to selfless action completed with love.

MANTRA YOGA – the path of sacred sound; the most sacred yoga mantra is the single syllable 'OM'.

HATHA YOGA – the path of physical control; regarded as a preparation for the pursuit of Raja Yoga. Hatha is the yoga form most widely practised in the West employing a combination of physical postures, breathing exercises, cleansing processes and awareness to prepare for contemplation and meditation.

RAJA YOGA OR 'ROYAL YOGA' – the path to enlightenment. The sage Patanjali defined this eight-step path in 200BC in his Yoga Sutras, an instruction manual for a full and productive life:

YAMA – a set of standards for ethical behaviour and social conduct

NIYAMA – self-discipline or individual conduct

ASANA – the practise of postures

PRANAYAMA – breath control

PRATYAHARA – sensory withdrawal (focusing the senses on the internal intellectual and spiritual world rather than the external social and physical world)

DHARANA – concentration

DHYANA – meditation

SAMADHI – the super-conscious state leading to self-realisation and the union of the soul with the Divine. The yogic concept of energy is prana, a life-force that operates within every living thing. The Chinese call this 'chi' and chart its flow through channels called meridians (similar to the Indian nadis); the Japanese call it 'ki' and believe that it resides in the abdomen. We can absorb prana by eating, drinking and breathing and can obtain it from sunshine, wind and rain. It is the vital energy that sustains life. At specific points along the midline of the body there are energy centres known as chakras. These are vibrational zones that carry information about all our organs and emotions and it is through them that the life-force energy flows to the rest of the body. Yoga prescribes asana, pranayama and kirya (cleansing exercises described in Stillness, see pages 94–5) to develop awareness of the chakras, clear the nadis and positively influence the flow of prana.

Benefits such as increased flexibility and calm may be noticed early on in yoga practice whilst others appear more slowly as new mind and body awareness is cultivated. Other physical benefits include increased strength, suppleness and stamina, and enhanced balance, posture, agility and grace. Regular practice can help to alleviate stress, insomnia, pre-menstrual tension, irritable bowel syndrome, headache, backache and asthma.

The internal systems and bodily processes are also cleansed and conditioned. The emphasis on breathing techniques helps the breath to become deeper and more full. This leads to clarity and stillness of mind that in turn enhances concentration. The benefits of improved health, fitness and concentration are well documented and now many forward-thinking schools are beginning to teach yoga to children. This has been shown to enhance self-confidence, academic performance and the ability to cope with stressful situations such as exams.

Yoga has become important in the lives of many contemporary Westerners not only as a way of improving health and fitness, but also as a means of personal and spiritual development. Religious beliefs have dwindled and as a result we often feel spiritually lost in the modern, industrialised world. Yoga offers a secular practice that can also meet our spiritual needs.

yoga

By opening the channels that connect the mind and spirit with the physical body, yoga helps to free stored emotions. You may experience dramatic emotions during or after performing postures or breathing exercises; do not be alarmed if you find yourself temporarily tearful, angry or frightened. Yoga does require detailed self-analysis but this is very different from demoralising self-criticism; it is not about success or failure but about personal development.

hatha yoga

Asana practice (yoga postures) can be hugely beneficial for everyone regardless of age, background, beliefs, lifestyle or physical and mental state. Continued asana practise gives strength and flexibility to muscular, skeletal and nervous systems. It promotes a healthy spine, massages and improves blood supply to internal organs, and improves circulation, digestion, elimination and respiration. The best introduction to asana practice is through classes that are taught by an experienced teacher. You need very few props: a yoga mat, a folded blanket and a foam or wooden block for support and, if you are stiff in the lower back or hamstring, a yoga strap to assist with stretches. Wear comfortable clothes that allow freedom of movement and go barefoot. Leave one hour after a light snack and at least three hours after a heavy meal before you undertake asana practice. You should adapt your asana practice to your own unique needs and lifestyle, particularly if you have a medical condition, an injury or if you are pregnant. Work out what it is that you would like to experience in yoga – spiritual discipline, muscle toning, injury recovery, flexibility or relaxation – and try different classes until you find one that meets your needs. Look for a teacher who gives clear instructions, corrects your postures on a one-on-one basis and responds readily to any questions. Within the discipline of Hatha yoga there are several teaching styles:

IYENGAR YOGA focuses on the precise physical alignment of each posture. Students learn asana first and then progress to breathing techniques.

ASHTANGA VINYASA YOGA each is a series of postures in a particular order. Students begin with the primary series, progress to the second series and finally to the advanced series. Postures are linked by a movement (vinyasa) to create a smooth, flowing sequence. Ashtanga Vinyasa is dynamic and physically demanding and uses a strong breathing technique (ujjayi, see page 119). A class that is advertised as 'Mysore-style practice' is for students who already know the series of postures.

DYNAMIC YOGA is a strong, flowing practice similar to ashtanga vinyasa but the postures are not taught in a series.

JIVAMUKTI YOGA has developed from ashtanga vinyasa. It is strong and dynamic and is characterised by spiritual teaching, chanting, breathing, meditation and a flowing sequence of postures.

BIKRAM'S YOGA teaches students a sequence of 26 postures in a room heated to more than 100 degrees Fahrenheit to rid the body of toxins and increase flexibility.

SIVANANDA YOGA comprises 12 basic postures and their variations, spiritual teaching, breathing techniques and chanting.

BIHAR YOGA, like Sivananda, is not physically demanding and may include spiritual or philosophical teaching.

VINI YOGA is a gentle form of yoga that includes breathing and posture practice as well as spiritual and philosophical teaching.

self-practice

Although you will learn a great deal from a teacher when starting out you will experience most of yoga's benefits by practising alone. Yoga is a process of self-realisation and you are the best expert on yourself.

Start developing self-practice at home to give yourself the opportunity to integrate what you have learnt in a class with your personal understanding of your body.

balance

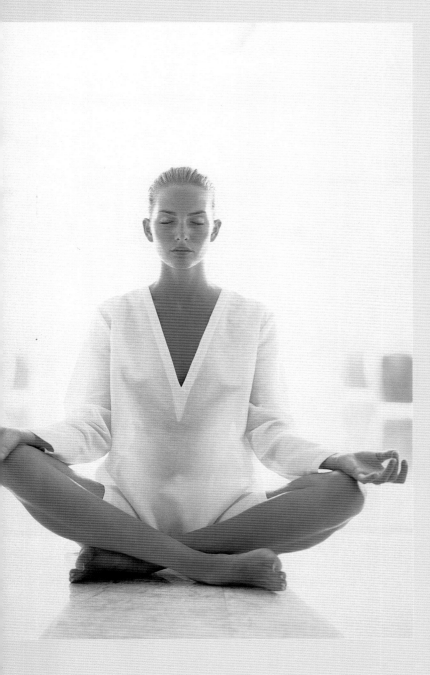

The two main obstacles to self-practice are discipline and self-confidence. Remember that yoga should be enjoyable and life enhancing. Start with postures that you feel confident about and use props to support you in a pose. Practising a variety of postures in sequence gives a balanced structure to your practise – choose sequences that suit your mood and energy levels. Try something dynamic and energising when you wake up in the morning and something relaxing after work; when physically exhausted use meditation techniques instead of postural practice. A little yoga practised often is far better than no yoga at all. Practise in a warm, clear space. Start with 15 minutes of practice 3 to 5 days a week, increasing to 45-minute sessions after a few months, aiming eventually for an hour or more daily with one rest day per week.

Be gentle with yourself. If you experience pain or pinching in any part of your body exit the pose slowly, consider what you are doing to produce the pain and modify your practice accordingly. Muscular discomfort can occur when you deepen into a posture and this should be embraced rather than resisted. Use your breath to develop a posture, grounding yourself on the in-breath and releasing your body further on each out-breath. The working loose of muscular tension is ultimately a healing process. As you practise asana your body yields or resists in various ways and feels different every day. This is yoga at work, bringing awareness and connection with your inner self.

All aspects of yoga are subtly interrelated and benefits gradually reveal themselves through continued practise. Through postural practise concentration and self-discipline develop. Breathing exercises give movement and life to the postures and help to improve meditative skills. Regular yoga practise creates a better quality of life.

bodywork

Therapeutic manipulation of the body is possibly the oldest of all healing traditions; no technological breakthrough can take the place of touch. Bodywork promotes good circulation and the release of muscular tension, promoting healing of stressed and injured tissue and better overall health. The reconnection of mind to body and of our senses to one another is the essence of bodywork. When we receive a massage in a candlelit room, with soft music playing and the scent of essential oils and a complementary tisane to sip afterwards, we are integrated living beings.

As bodywork is one-on-one, time intensive and involves touch it can seem very personal and to some intimidating or self-indulgent. However, no-one can deny the restorative power of treatments and the positive effect of another's undivided attention focused on our personal wellbeing. Touch is our most basic form of communication: it lets us know we are not alone; it soothes and reassures us.

swedish massage is the basis from which many other Western massage techniques have been developed. It dates back to the 1830s and is a brisk, vigorous full-body massage employing a combination of long strokes and kneading in the direction of the heart. The emphasis is on increasing circulation in the surface muscles using five basic strokes:

EFFLEURAGE – smooth gliding strokes used to relax soft tissues, usually applied with both hands.

FRICTION – the deepest stroke, which causes underlying layers of tissue to rub against each other, increasing blood flow, breaking up adhesions and freeing muscle fibres.

PETRISSAGE – a pulsating motion that involves squeezing, rolling and kneading muscles.

TAPOTEMENT – a rapid, rhythmic tapping to stimulate the nerves.

COMPRESSION – rhythmic, pump-like pressure that promotes movement of the blood and the lymph through tissues.

deep tissue massage is slow and focused to flush out soft tissue, release chronic muscle tension and break up adhesions or calcified bruises in the muscles.

sports massage is useful for anyone with chronic pain, injury or range-of-motion issues and the work is usually limited to a specific area.

lymphatic drainage massage uses very light, rhythmic strokes to stimulate and promote the movement of lymphatic fluids.

aromatherapy couples therapeutic massage with specially customised essential oils to enhance the healing benefits of touch.

la stone therapy glides heated basalt stones over the body to simultaneously relax and stimulate the muscles.

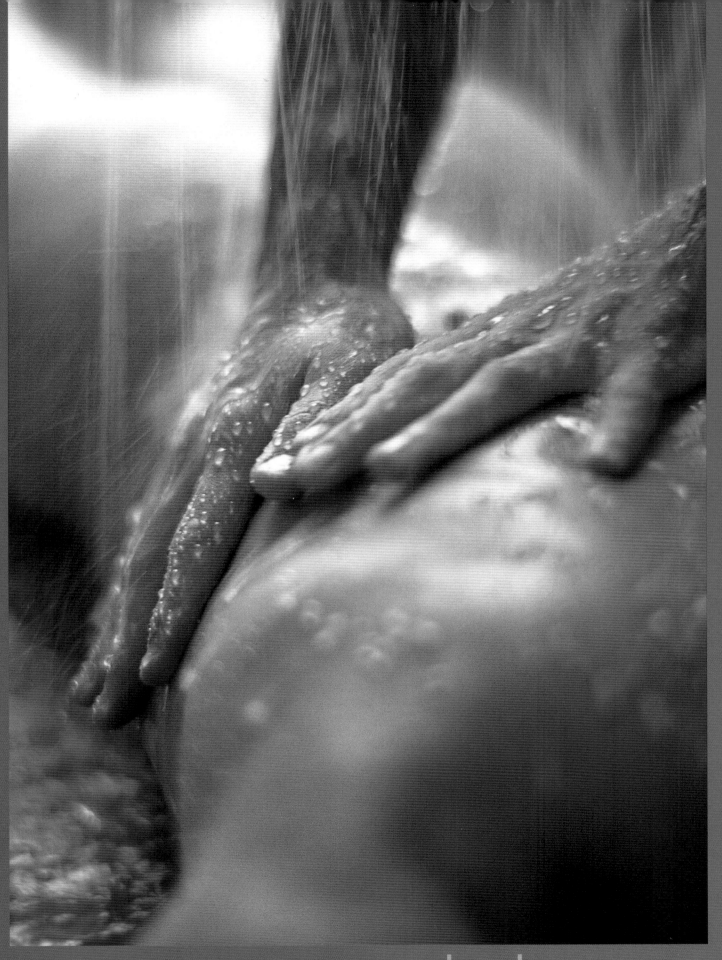

balance

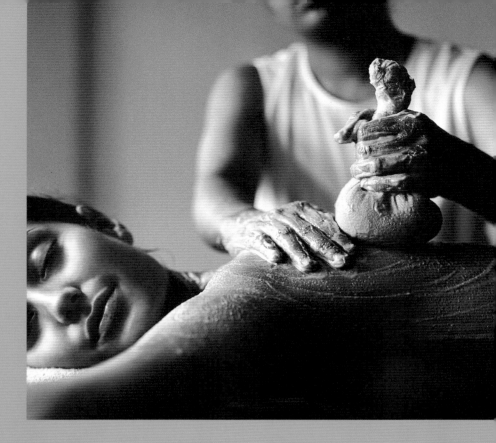

eastern bodywork techniques

Eastern therapies stem from the idea of energy flow that runs through the body along channels or meridians. The aim of the treatment is to balance and regulate the energy in the body. Herbs, colour therapy and aromatherapy are sometimes combined with these methods.

acupuncture is one of the oldest forms of natural healing. Fine needles are inserted into the energy channels just under the surface of the skin to help re-direct the flow of chi and restore the balance and state of harmony.

shiatsu involves applying finger pressure to acupuncture points for the purposes of balancing the flow of chi.

reflexology has much in common with shiatsu and acupressure, and involves stimulation of specific points on the hands and feet that correspond to organs, glands, systems and parts of the body. With the aid of a reflexology chart and patience you can effectively massage yourself.

jin shin jyutsu is a very gentle form of treatment that uses pulse diagnosis to identify and release blockages in the flow of chi.

thai massage uses a variety of stretching and rocking movements that apply pressure to the body's energy points to loosen tight muscles and increase the range of motion. This style of bodywork is revitalising for both mind and body and accelerates rehabilitation by effectively relieving joint tension and reducing muscle recovery time.

tui na is a physical, and physically demanding, form of Chinese medical massage undertaken only after a lengthy diagnostic process. Skin texture, colour, pulse, tongue and emotional state are considered as well as the symptoms. Pressure is applied using the practitioner's hands, fingers and elbows and various stretches are performed.

ayurvedic treatments

Designed to balance and nourish the body, mind and spirit, Ayurvedic treatments begin with an identification of the individual's physical type and condition. These therapies emphasise the use of fragrance, colour and touch in a variety of soothing treatments. Ayurveda encompasses regulation of diet, sleep, physical activity and cleansing treatments. We are born with our own individual constitutions and how we treat our bodies, minds and spirits affects their balance. What is beneficial for one individual may be detrimental to another; exercises that promote wellbeing in one may increase stress in another. Our daily routines should be tailored accordingly to find our own perfect balance.

Ayurveda is one of the world's oldest fully integrated healing systems. It assesses what is required on all levels to be in balance and to create harmony both within ourselves and between ourselves and our environment. When we are out of balance we become susceptible to stress and subsequently disease. In Ayurvedic medicine the human body is composed of the five elements, air, fire, water, earth and space, which are the basic building blocks of everything in the universe. There are three main body types or doshas: vata (space and air), pitta (fire) and kapha (earth and water). While we all manifest characteristics of all three doshas we tend to lean more towards one or two of them from birth. An Ayurvedic-trained doctor will diagnose your dominant dosha, identify imbalances and give you dietary advice, a prescription of herbal remedies, exercise recommendations, breathing techniques and therapeutic massage.

ABHYANGA MASSAGE involves two therapists using warm Ayurvedic oils in synchronisation to expel tension and accumulated toxins from the body. These oils are tailored to the individual client's dosha or body type.

INDIAN HEAD MASSAGE works with firm rhythms to release blockages in the neck and shoulders where tension is particularly prone to accumulate. The scalp and underlying muscles are worked on to relieve headaches and eyestrain, inducing a state of revitalised calm.

PANCHAKARMA is an intensive detox programme usually combining fasting and colonic irrigation with other Ayurvedic therapies.

SHIRODHARA is a balancing massage focusing on the energy points or marmas on the face, neck and upper chest, and the chakra points on the body, to release tension. It is especially effective for those experiencing anxiety, stress, insomnia and depression. Oils are chosen to suit your dosha, and a steady stream of warmed oil is continuously poured onto the centre of your forehead that helps instil a profound sense of relaxation in the furthermost corners of the mind.

In our modern world we are beginning to understand that stress-relief and increased wellbeing are essential for a happy, healthy life. The myriad of therapies now available to us testify to this change in attitude. Some therapies are based on the idea of a surrounding universal energy that can be channelled by the practitioner, including reiki, which is non-tactile, and polarity therapy, in which the practitioner uses gentle touch. Others therapies have been developed to answer a specific need. Craniosacral therapy detects and treats problems of the skull, spinal column and sacrum. Applied kinesiology uses muscle reaction to test physical imbalances such as food intolerance. To prevent and treat illness and increase vitality, homeopathy and flower remedies use natural substances, while naturopathy combines diet, osteopathy and hydrotherapy. Other elements also now being used as therapies include crystals to direct energy at specific problems, colour for enhanced wellbeing, and light for depression and low energy levels. Find the therapy that works for you and book yourself in for a treatment whenever you feel the need.

balance

detox diet

Some people find that having incorporated asana practice and pranayama into their lives they want to broaden their yoga practice to include the principles of social and personal conduct, which naturally leads them to the yogic diet. Asana practice can encourage a heightened awareness of the effect of meat and substances such as caffeine and alcohol on the mind and body. You may also find that asana practice sharpens your sense of taste and smell, reducing cravings for sugary, spicy and salty food.

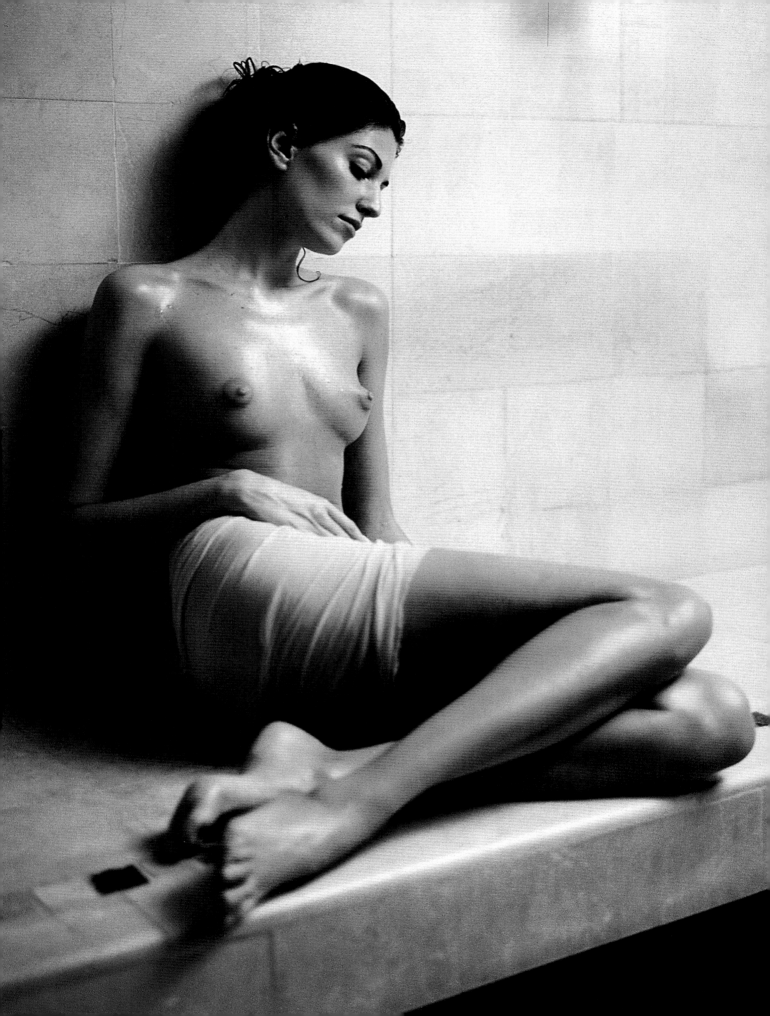

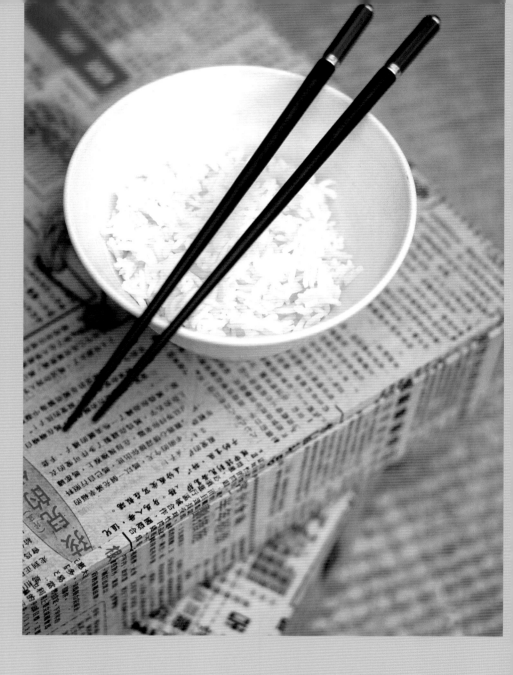

Eating a balanced, lacto-vegetarian, organic diet helps to keep the body slender and improves flexibility and physical wellbeing. With a rational of 'ahimsa', or non-harm to all living things, **the yogic diet helps clear and focus the mind,** and contains all the necessary elements to sustain, heal and develop the body without burdening it with excess toxins.

The yogic diet is made up entirely of non-animal foods, with the exceptions of milk, cheese, yoghurt, butter, eggs and honey, and foods are eaten in their natural state as much as possible. Processed and convenience foods, white flour, sugar, foods that contain colouring, added sugar or salt, and modified starches or fats are

avoided. Yoga does not demand overnight conversions or changes in lifestyle; eating more vegetarian meals week by week will allow your body time to adjust.

Water accounts for around 70 per cent of the human body mass and is vital to its functioning. Without water we cannot effectively eliminate toxins and waste matter or grow new tissue. Never try to lose weight by cutting down on the amount of water you drink. Drinking plenty of water can sometimes overcome weight problems and fluid retention that is often due to a toxic or mineral imbalance in the body. By increasing the amount of water you drink this imbalance may be resolved. To get into the habit of drinking more water drink a glass every hour from the time you wake up until the time you go to sleep. Another way is to drink as much as you can first thing in the morning, which is quite easy if you have exercised first thing, and then smaller amounts throughout the day.

You can increase your overall intake of fluids by drinking herbal teas, fruit and vegetable juices, and by eating water-rich foods such as fruit and vegetables. Citrus fruits, green leafy vegetables, melons, apricots and avocado are also full of vitamin C, calcium and the B group of vitamins (B1, B6, folic acid and pantothenic acid). These nutrients are known to have a tranquillising, balancing effect on the nervous system and can be effective in stress relief. Experiment with some calming juice combinations such as black-currant and apple, or carrot, celery and mangetout.

Fasting is an extremely effective way to cleanse the body and purify the mind. A fast allows the entire digestive system time to rest and this energy is instead used to repair and strengthen the body's systems.

Fasting can make people feel particularly alert and clear-headed, enabling them to focus better and achieve longer periods of meditation. It is an act of self-discipline that must be carefully managed and should only be used to cleanse the system and restore balance to the body, not to lose weight.

A short fast can last between one and three days. A one-day fast can rest the digestive system but a longer fast is required for the body to undergo full detoxification. As fasting involves some disruption to your everyday life, plan to fast during a period when you do not have to work and are able to devote your time to rest. A gentle practice of yoga postures can, however, speed up the process of detoxification.

Two days before a fast prepare your body by simplifying your diet to a few basic ingredients: fruit, vegetables and perhaps some yoghurt. On the day of your fast eliminate all solid foods and only drink either fruit or vegetable juice, remembering not to mix the two in the same glass. Drink about 4 litres of juice a day and try to 'chew' it rather than simply gulping it down as this aids digestion.

During a fast toxins and impurities are released from the body through all the organs of elimination including the skin. Wash regularly to keep the skin fresh and clean and try body brushing to help remove dead skin cells and stimulate the circulatory, lymph and nervous systems. As the body goes through its internal cleaning process you may experience skin eruptions, which should clear up in a few days. It is completely normal to feel a little cold and shivery while fasting so make sure you dress warmly. Other side effects include headaches, bad breath, a coated tongue, dizziness, mild palpitations and nausea. However, should you experience any breathing difficulties or strong palpita-tions immediately seek the advice of a doctor.

On the last evening of a fast eat one type of fresh fruit, avoiding acidic fruits such as oranges. The following morning around 10am eat some more fruit and perhaps a small bowl of yoghurt. Have a similar meal around 5pm. The next day your diet should consist of raw vegetables and salads, and the following day you can add rice or another grain and some steamed vegetables. After this you can continue eating normally.

escape

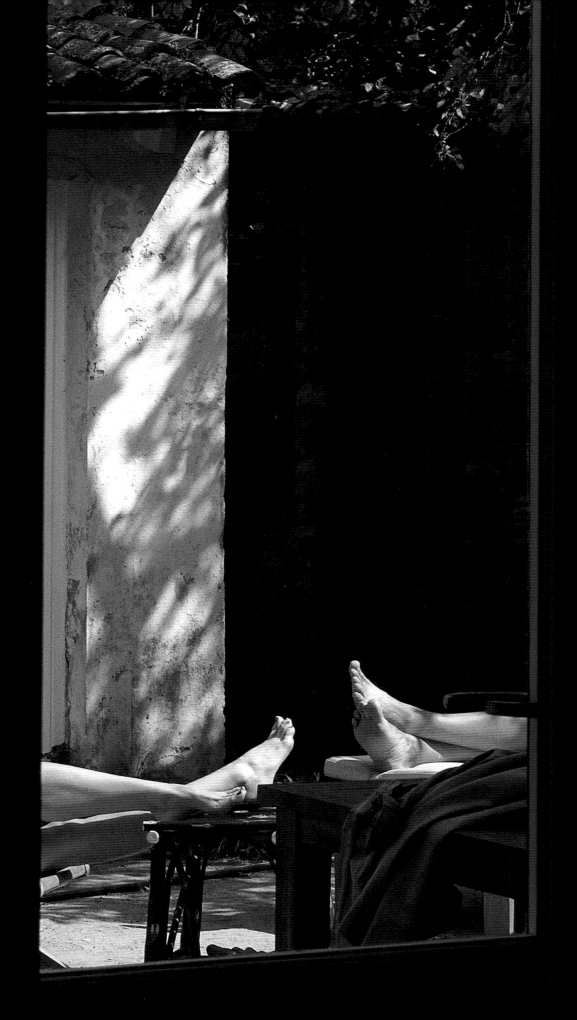

escape

Escape is an essential stop on the curative road to wellbeing. Time away from the daily grindstone is extraordinarily beneficial to the mind, body and soul. It is easy to believe that we can't afford to take time out from work, but in reality we function more effectively when our batteries have been recharged. Breaks taken little and often can be as beneficial as a longer holiday; how you employ your time will determine how uplifting and lasting its effect.

Escape is 'time for me', doing something that fills the heart with happiness. It could be as simple as taking half a day off to visit some galleries or perhaps watching movies back-to-back in an art house cinema. More often it involves the great outdoors and a soul-inspiring sense of adventure: driving to a favourite beach to walk along the windswept shores; mountain biking off-road to explore a new woodland trail; an invigorating weekend of sailing. Fresh air loaded with negative ions brings radiance to the cheeks and a spring to our step; the sounds, sights and scents of the natural world refresh the senses and liberate the mind.

A sun-drenched holiday is often our chosen form of escape, but we do not have to travel a long way to get the benefits of a break from the norm. Plan a trip to a local day spa, choosing treatments that invigorate and detox you, relax and revive you. The possibilities are endless. Your imagination and your pocket are the only limiting factors and, if necessary, most treatments can be substituted by DIY versions in the comfort of your own home. Self-indulgent time out is one of life's essentials that should not be ignored. Cherish the feeling in your body after your treatment; remind yourself that every nerve in your being is alive.

Stress accumulates and from time to time we need to do something a little more radical to remove stresses and toxins. In this instance a retreat can be immensely beneficial, taking us away from our regular environment to a quieter place for contemplation and detoxification. This can vary from a relaxing weekend away to a remote place specialising in physical, mental or spiritual cleansing. Spend time at an ashram or, at the other end of the spectrum, visit an exclusive destination spa totally dedicated to relaxation and pampering. Savour every moment of your experience: take time to listen to your body and calm your mind; take delight in feeding your body healthy, fresh, enticing foods; relax and unwind in your peaceful, serene surroundings.

energising escape

One of the most effective ways to restore your equilibrium and give your body and mind a break is to take part in a sporting activity or outdoor pursuit. To push yourself physically beyond your own expectations is to open your eyes to possibility. Regular exercise not only increases your level of fitness but also boosts your self-confidence; you know that the benefits you get are a direct result of the hard work you put in and you can revel in your achievements. Learn to love the feeling of working your body hard, and take pleasure in all the beneficial effects of the after-exercise glow.

For an energising and fun way to take time out make full use of your local gym, or your gym membership, and plan an activity weekend with a friend. Try an assortment of classes each day, perhaps starting with an early-morning yoga or stretch class. Then move onto a cardio workout or go spinning, following that with a swim, use of the hydrotherapy pool and a steam or sauna. Enjoy spending time with your friend and encourage each other to keep motivated during every class. You could book yourself a La Stone-therapy or deep-tissue massage to help work the toxins out of the body, and a manicure or pedicure to reward yourself after your efforts.

If you would prefer to take your exercise out of doors there are legions of activities just waiting to be explored. Learn to horse-back ride at the nearest coast to your home so that you can canter through the surf just like they do in the movies. Play a round of golf with your friends or just go onto the driving range and release your stress and tension by thwacking a few balls as far as you can. Book an activity holiday to learn a new skill or improve a neglected one: try tennis camp, windsurfing school or water-skiing classes. Take a weekend break to the mountains and go rock-climbing or skiing, or to the coast for surfing or hiking. Revel in your surroundings while you are pushing yourself to extremes. Write a diary or take photographs to remind you of the inspirational moments of your time; looking back on an enjoyable break can bring its own uplifting rewards. Think about the places and pursuits that give you most pleasure and then find a way to get out there and do what makes you happy.

escape

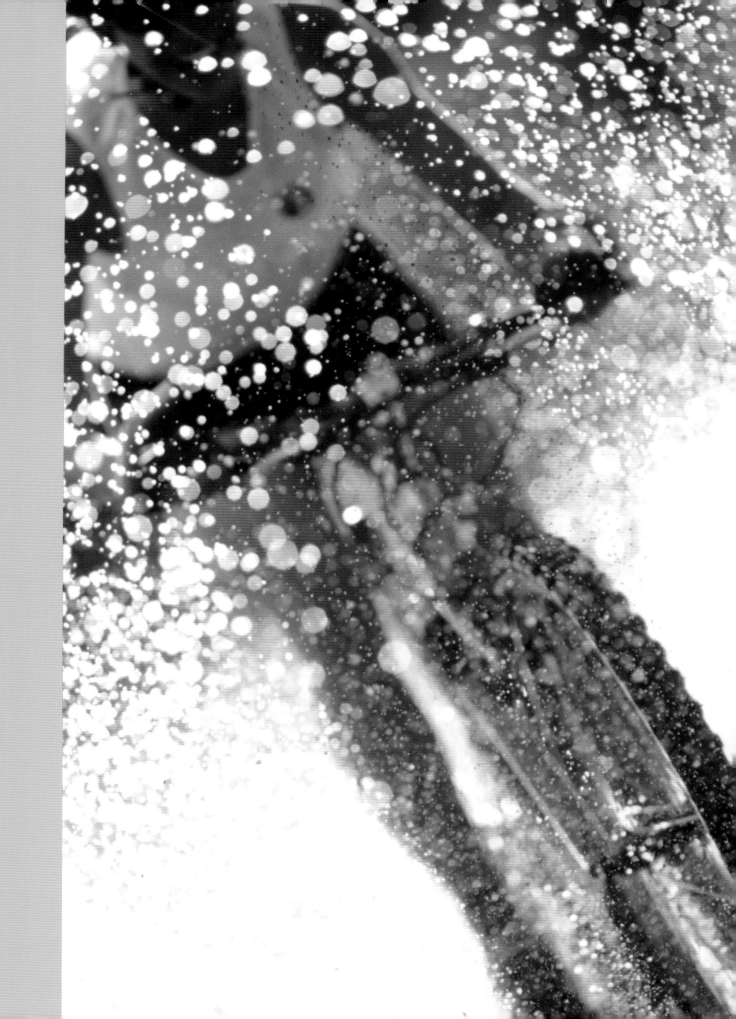

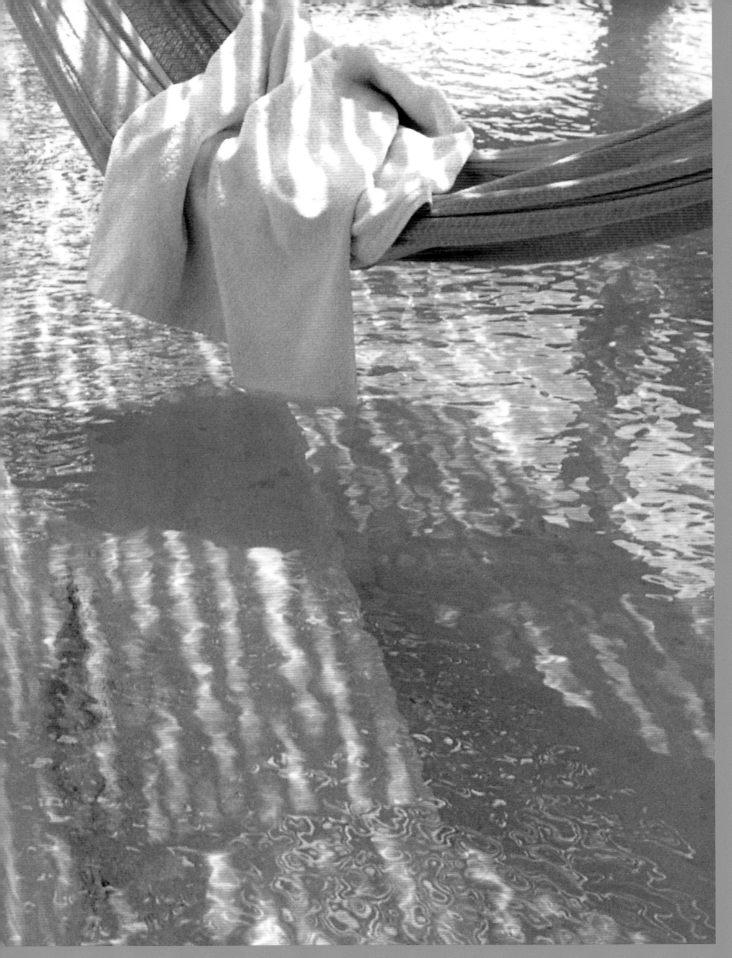

escape

holiday hideaway

Your ideal escape may be to a beautiful beach in an exotic locale: soaking up the rays while floating in a sea of blue can bring body, mind and soul together. However, travelling can be uncomfortable and tiring, which is not what you want on a relaxing break, so take a little time to look after yourself.

When flying follow a few sensible precautions to increase your comfort. Drink plenty of still water and avoid caffeine and alcohol. Remove make-up and apply a hydrating moisturiser and eye cream. Regularly apply lip balm and spray your face with an aromatic herbal spritzer. Wear glasses rather than contact lenses or take some solution with you. Reduce your risk of 'economy class syndrome' or Deep Vein Thrombosis (DVT): before you fly take an aspirin to thin your blood; during the flight wear compression socks and boost your circulation by stretching and moving your body.

To relieve symptoms of travel sickness use an acupressure travel band or chew on crystallised ginger or the herb angelica. Before you leave home blend 2 drops of peppermint essential oil with a little sweet almond oil and rub into your chest. To limit the effects of jet lag, eat and sleep according to the time of your destination while you are on the plane and take a walk as soon as you arrive.

One of the reasons we love a beach-resort holiday is the resulting tan. A tan can boost our confidence and make us feel more attractive, but in reality the only safe tan is a fake tan. New tanning products offer scent-free, natural colour without the damaging effects of lengthy sun exposure, but remember that a fake tan offers absolutely no sun protection so all the usual sunscreen rules apply.

Always use a high SPF sunscreen (at least factor 15) that includes UVA and UVB protection: UVA rays speed up ageing, damage elasticity and increase the long-term risk of skin cancer; UVB rays cause sunburn and redness. Make sure your sunscreen includes either titanium dioxide (good on sensitive skins) or zinc oxide, both of which block UVA and UVB rays, or a combination of avobenzone (Parsol) a UVA filter and octyl-methoxycinnimate (OMC), a UVB filter.

Apply your sunscreen at least 20 minutes before going out into the sun and reapply every 1–2 hours and immediately after swimming. Drink plenty of water to prevent dehydration. Only sunbathe in short bursts before 11am and after 3pm. Do not expose babies under six months to the sun and take extra care with children. Do not wear alcohol-based perfume or acne preparations (e.g. benzoyl peroxide) in the sun, or expose recently waxed or shaved skin, as irritation can occur. Remember that the sun can dry out your hair so wear a hat or use a special hair sunscreen. As soon as you return indoors cool down with a tepid bath or shower and moisturise the skin well.

destination spas

When you take a break away it is foolish not to come back in better shape than when you left, which is why spas have become so popular in recent years. A spa vacation is an investment in yourself; it will get your body back in motion and teach you about healthy nutrition and meaningful recreation for the mind as well as for the body.

The destination spa concept has moved on from the old European spa where the elderly elite went to take the waters and be attended to by doctors. Now many destination spas offer specific programmes to cleanse and tone the body, relax the mind and nurture the spirit. They offer the perfect escape from our high-tech, 24/7 lifestyles so that we can benefit from the meditative lifestyle of serenity. Spas emphasise many different benefits and treatments: holistic health, life enhancement, luxury pampering, nutrition and diet, weight management, preventive medicine, spiritual awareness, sports conditioning, stress control and taking the waters. They all strive to help each one of us to be the best that we can be at the things we most care about.

A retreat or spa vacation is one of the few holidays where the greatest benefit is derived by going alone. Loneliness is never an issue since other hardworking people seeking healthy turnarounds make wonderful companions. In the supportive environment of health resorts, guests as well as staff soon develop more than customary concern for one another's welfare. The general feeling is one of 'we're all in this together'.

Decide whether you are looking to relax amid the elite in a luxury resort or whether you will find gratification in the more rugged atmosphere of a ranch with a rigorous 'boot camp' schedule. First you have to choose between the self-contained spa or retreat that focuses on wellness, and resorts that feature a spa or health club along with sports and other diversions. In the wellness programmes you will find group support and camaraderie from like-minded participants who are also adhering to the structured daily schedule. At the resorts you may be more self-indulgent, as there are many options and temptations geared towards those who are on a non-spa holiday. Choice made, you then have to decide the form of programme from which you will derive greatest benefit.

escape

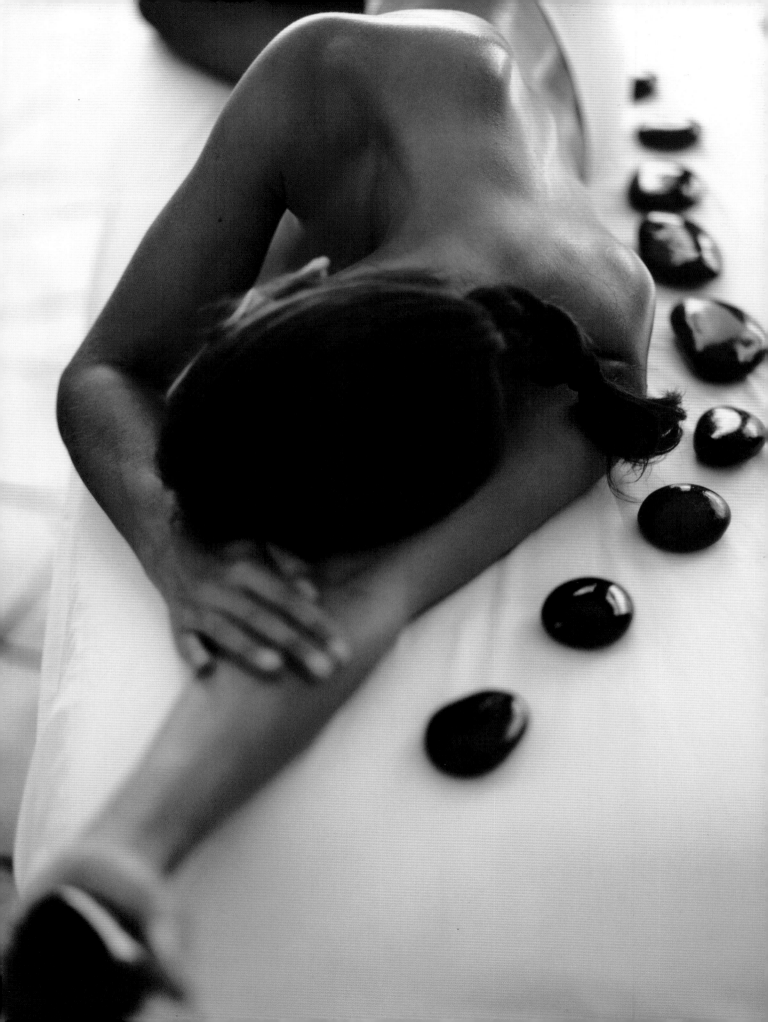

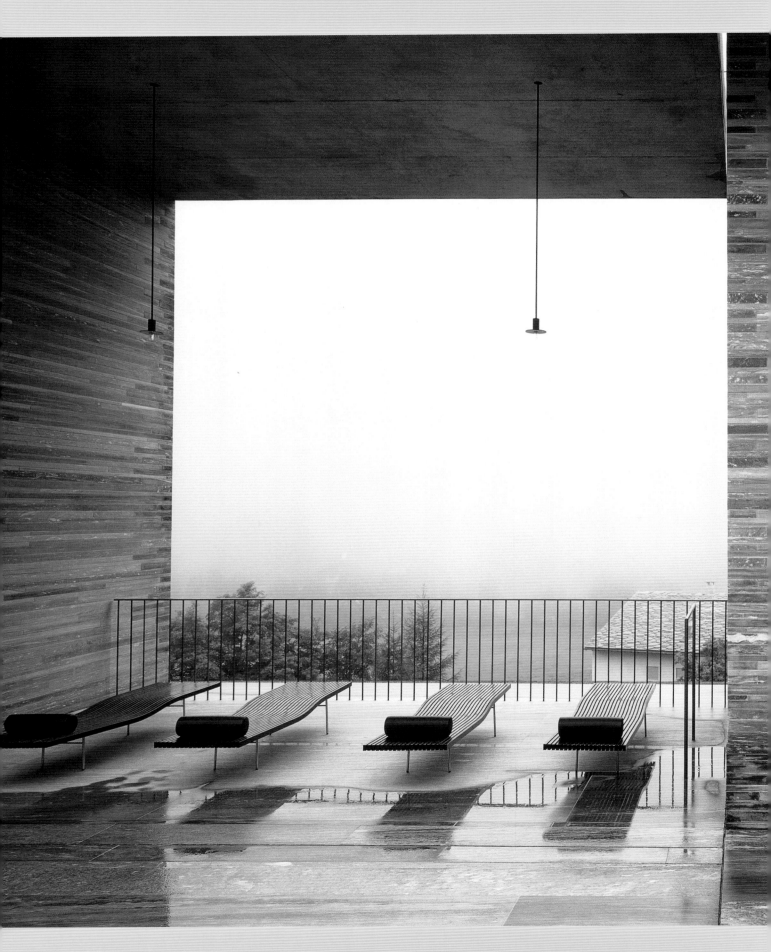

spiritual retreats

New Age retreats and yoga ashrams, naturopaths and natural healing centres offer health and healing based on combinations of ancient therapies and the latest concepts in behaviour modification. Some establishments preach preventive medicine, taking a holistic approach toward strengthening the body against illness through improved nutrition and an understanding of the relationship between mind and body. Others address such problems as the need to lose weight, to stop smoking and to deal with stress. These programmes educate participants, reinforce motivation and provide a regimen designed not for quick results but for effective long-term improvement in wellbeing. They help guests change their lifestyles at home.

The credo of holistic health retreats is that illness results from a lack of balance within the body, whether caused by stress or physical conditions,and that balance can be restored without the use of medicine. The premise is that in order to be truly fit and healthy the emotional, intellectual and spiritual self must be developed as well as the body. Non-traditional therapies are used to achieve a sense of wholeness with the world and oneself that boosts the body's immune system. In celebrating human potential, spiritual-awareness programmes strive to stretch the individual's limits both mentally and physically. They try to foster a process of personal growth and transformation through workouts that synchronise mind and body. Specialising in alternative education, vegetarian diets and natural therapies, holistic programmes suggest that by raising awareness of our inner resources we can counteract and reduce stress.

Holistic health training can be vigorous or mellow with a combination of exercise, nutrition, stress control and relaxation. The experience may draw on any number of Eastern and Western philosophies and healing processes including yogic training, sensory awareness, body therapies, visualisation or shamanism. Meditation is also taught extensively. Retreats rather than resorts, these centres for spiritual training are situated in places where nature's beauty can be enjoyed without distraction or tension. When undertaken in a secluded place of great natural beauty, the healing process may draw on spiritual sources as well as natural energy to help participants find inner strength.

Life-enhancement programmes aim for long-term physical and psychological benefits. They involve a complete health assessment with medical tests and personal consultations on nutrition and fitness. Some programmes have a spiritual element whilst others emphasise an educational approach through exercise, diet and behaviour modification. Such programmes require total commitment from the participants.Group sizes are small and everyone works on a one-to-one basis with the health and behavioural specialists in an intensive experience that little resembles a resort-style programme.

Preventive medicine centres combine traditional medical services with advanced concepts for the prevention of illness. A regenerative experience, the programmes involve health and fitness testing, counselling on nutrition and stress control, and a range of sports and exercise activities along with massage and bodywork. Participants work with a team of physiotherapists and doctors to learn how to eliminate negative habits and modify a lifestyle for survival. One-on-one training with fitness instructors, nutritionists and psychologists reveals how personal goals can be accomplished.

health programmes

The increasing ageing population has resulted in health and fitness programmes designed specifically for men and women over the age of 50. Combining elements of spa vacations with medical services and lifestyle education, these programmes promote a healthier way of working, exercising and eating. The emphasis is on preventing illness by staying fit.

Nutrition and diet programmes maintain that wellbeing begins in the kitchen, that understanding the relationship between nutrition and diet can enhance your lifestyle and promote sound, healthy habits. A new perspective is offered through lectures and first-hand experience in food preparation. Subjects covered include how foods affect your health, how to shop, how to choose from restaurant menus and how to plan and prepare meals. Designed as an educational experience the programme provides the fundamentals for following a regimen of eating healthy, natural foods.

Learning how to lose weight properly and how to maintain a healthy balance in body mass is the basis of weight-management programmes. These courses teach proper eating habits rather than offering dramatic weight loss. The weight-management resort integrates motivational sessions with exercise, diet with pampering, re-education with recreation. Some programmes involve fasting on juices and water. Carefully controlled and supervised, the typical regimen is tailored to the individual's fitness level and health needs.

luxury spas

At the other end of the spectrum are resorts that focus on luxury pampering – perfect for those who long to be herbal wrapped, massaged to a pulp and soaked in bubbling hydrotherapy pools. The height of survival chic is lounging in an elegant robe and discussing a delicious spa meal. Exercise classes and a weight-loss diet may form part of the treatment but are usually optional. The services include the latest image-enhancers at the beauty salon, herbal enzyme face peels, loofah body scrubs and salt rubs, aromatherapy massage, Ayurvedic therapies and paraffin pedicures, alongside underwater massage, hydrotherapy with thermal waters and thalassotherapy with seaweed products and seawater.

Mineral-rich, Dead Sea waters and mud have been credited for thousands of years with relieving certain forms of eczema and psoriasis and in particular the pain associated with arthritis. This is due to its very high concentration of potassium, calcium and magnesium, which soothe tissue.

Therapeutic mud and clays come in a variety of colours – yellow, white, green, black and brown – from sources such as Italy's Montecatini thermal springs, Rhassoul mud from Morocco, the Black Sea and the Dead Sea. Mud treatments are extremely detoxifying as they draw out surface debris from the skin; excess sebum, toxins and dead cells can then be rinsed away.

Therapies in which the body soaks in mineral- and algae-rich waters are standard cures in French Thalassotherapy centres. Sea bathing is an ancient ever-popular cure even if we now call it 'going to the beach'. Seawater is the most mineral-rich element in the world and oceanic plants concentrate these nutrients thousands of times. In addition, seaside air is loaded with negative ions, which makes us full of energy. In some spas hydrotherapy equipment is combined with mud and algae for body cleansing and the latest in toning, shaping and weight-loss techniques.

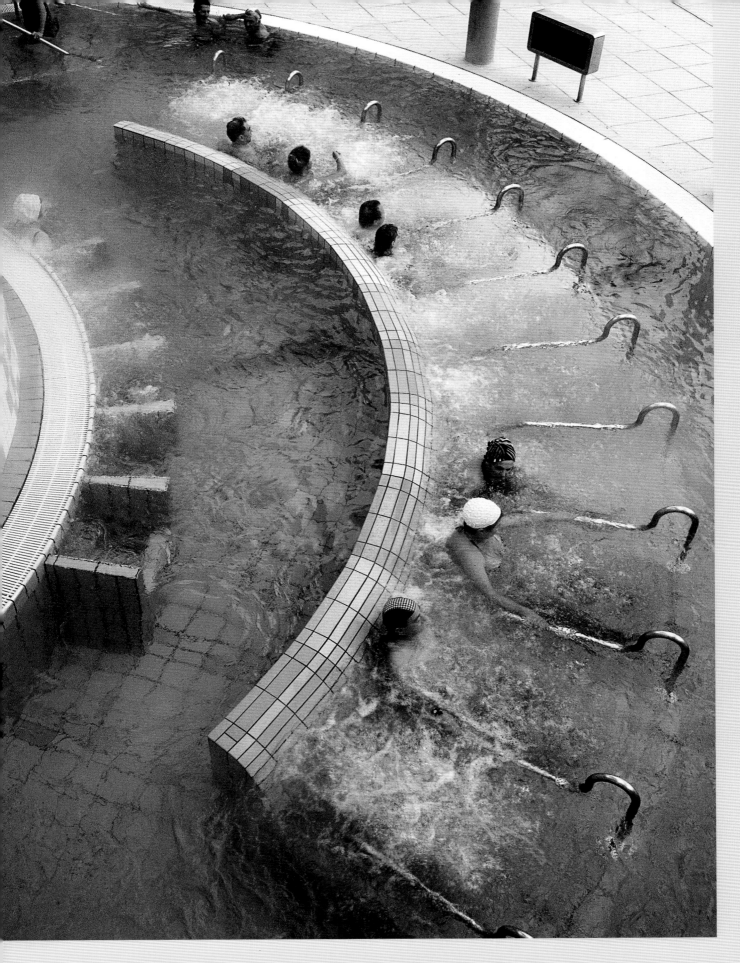

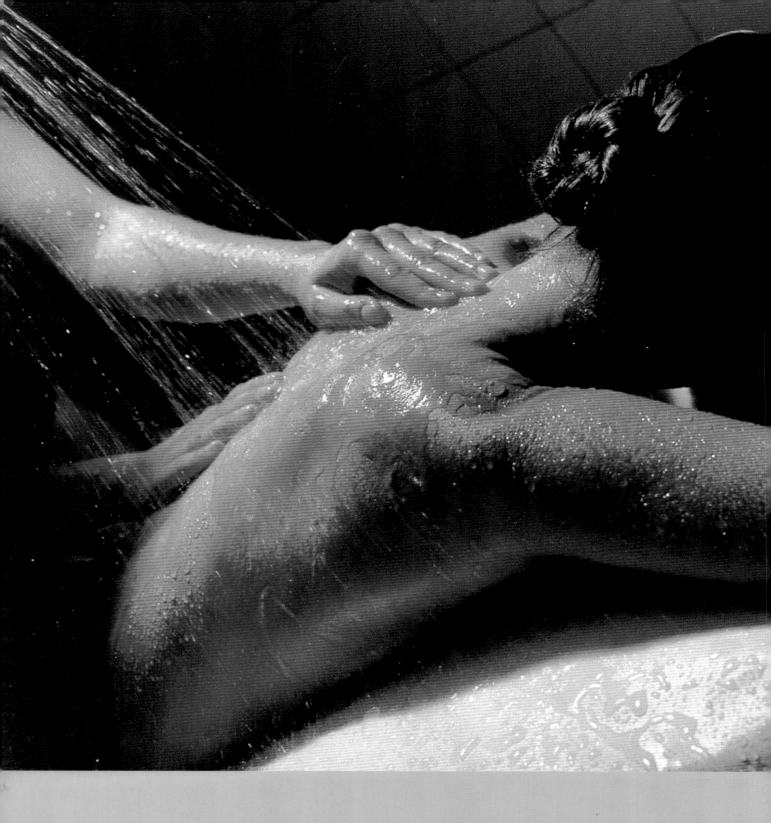

escape

day spas

Many of the more luxurious, pampering treatments are also available at day spas. If there are a few day spas in your area try to have a look around them all before booking your day of escape; each will offer different treatments and have an atmosphere all its own and you need to find one that feels special for you. Are you attracted by the hustle and bustle of a more social spa, one in which you can drink herbal tea in the lounge between treatments and talk to others around you, or do you need silence and peace to collect your thoughts and calm your soul?

To take full advantage of your day start off with an invigorating salt rub to thoroughly exfoliate the body top to toe, following that with a detox seaweed wrap to kick start the elimination processes. Then enjoy a deeply relaxing aromatherapy massage before ending the day with an aromatic, deep-cleansing facial.

Treat yourself; escape from your normal life for one day and book a few treatments that you've always wanted to experience. Soak up the ambience, enjoy indulging yourself and take pleasure in the attentiveness of each therapist. Allow thoughts of the world outside to drift away and revel in the peace and tranquillity you discover within yourself.

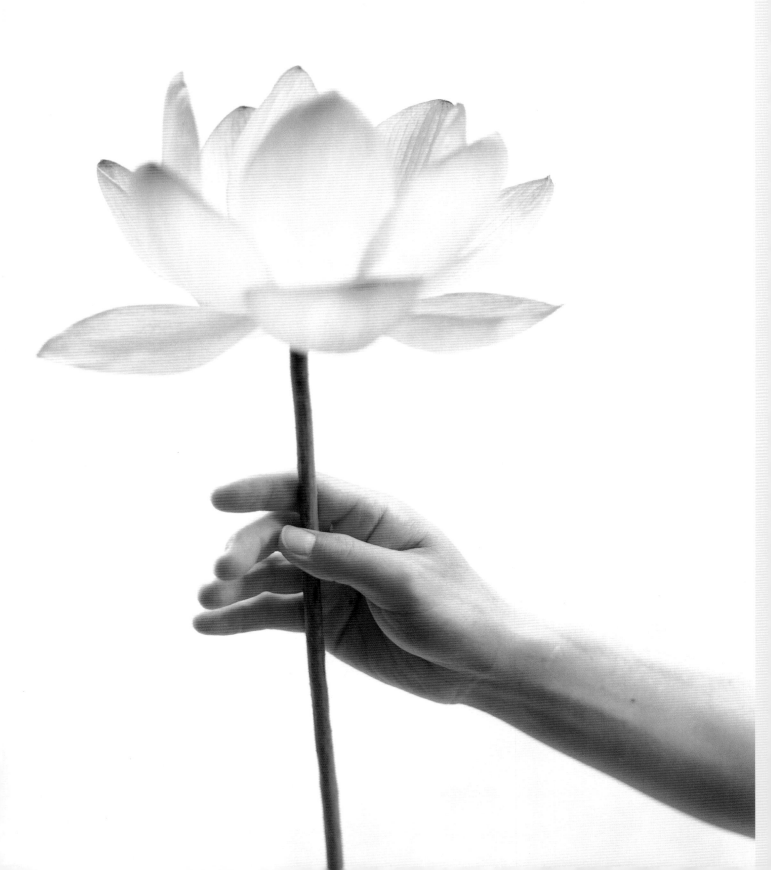

inspire

So what does the future hold? The consumer is becoming increasingly educated in terms of product choice, ingredients and their application. Accordingly there will be a rise in home customisation where the consumer can adapt her routine products to meet her changing daily demands, which she in turn is taking more time to actively define. This will produce an increase in specialist make-up: under-bases, primers, special-effects powders and glosses for both lips and eyes. From this comes deeper knowledge in application techniques that require greater discernment and appreciation of quality in make-up tools.

Skincare will continue to develop in two different directions: new high-tech formulations are appearing from Japan and the United States, while at the other end of the spectrum Europe is leading a return to more ritualistic, organic and plant-based solutions inspired by other cultures such as Ayurvedic, Native American Indian and Indonesian. People are becoming more focused on nutrition, vitamin and mineral supplementation. Skincare and haircare companies are beginning to market supplements to enhance their regular products, alongside the introduction of specialist complementary elixirs and teas.

The home spa industry is booming: a pampering night in is now a real alternative to a night on the town. We are slowly but surely becoming a nurturing culture. At long last beauty specialists are emerging in different fields, from bodywork and facials to manicures and eyebrow-shaping. The 'jack-of-all-trades' beauty therapist, who in the past has been expected to give a manicure one minute and offer a soul-nurturing deep-tissue massage the next (an impossible task in my view), will be a thing of the past. We are now seeing a global expectation of high standards. This is being driven by the increasingly well-travelled consumer who is experiencing treatments during vacations and is no longer prepared to compromise with second best at home. The consumer base is also growing as the massage treat on holiday develops into a weekly de-stressing ritual. Treatments are now using essential oils, coloured light, sound frequencies and poultices of herbs and algae – all sensory stimulants. There is no mystery as to why such treatments are effective: our senses are highways to the brain, which controls our biochemistry.

We are seeing similar extremes within the exercise industry. High-tech gym equipment is facing constant upgrade, with audio-visual evolution the subject of global trials after the success of spin classes. Body pump has taken weight training into the aerobics studio and in contrast yoga and Pilates mat-work classes are vying for studio time. Specialist yoga studios are de rigeur and tai chi, chi gong and meditation classes are their complements. Outdoor pursuits in the form of hiking and mountain biking are gaining in popularity and this partly stems from an unconscious desire to commune with nature.

inspire

Our increased awareness in wellbeing is promoting change within the workplace and at home. Designers are beginning to take the senses into account with increasing attention being paid to the impact of colour, form, materials and texture, coupled with ambient lighting, fragrance and music. Bathrooms are gaining in importance and being viewed as relaxation chambers. Home exercise areas are on the increase as are defined spaces for reflection and contemplation. Gardens are becoming an extension of the home with blurred boundaries between indoors and out. Along with a general interest in Eastern minimal aesthetics and philosophies, there are also influences from North Africa and Europe in colour palette and the use of aromatic plants. Globalisation, specialisation and customisation are recurrent themes in all areas of life.

Many of us live happily with the passage of time, while others turn to plastic surgeons in the unnatural quest for eternal youth. Age is more about attitude than grey hair or wrinkles. It is important to recognise the full potential of our lives. Look at life afresh, free from the delusions of ego, opinions and prejudice. With freedom of mind and spirit the ordinary becomes the extraordinary. We should learn to live compassionately and creatively and to take responsibility for ourselves and for all living things — all life is interconnected.

There are no guarantees in life — we all accept that. By creating a healthy, balanced life you are giving yourself the greatest possibility of living each day with vitality, joy, fulfilment and dignity. Never look back and say 'If only…'. As an old Chinese proverb says 'the journey of a thousand miles begins with a single step'. Lifestyle change is a project for the rest of your life and moving in the right direction is much more important than the speed at which you travel. Know where you stand right now, have a vision of where you want to go and, when you are ready, begin putting one foot in front of the other.

Open your eyes to the world that surrounds you.

Open your ears to the impact of music.

Open your mind to spiritual riches.   Savour the fruits that the earth can offer.

Succumb to the healing power of touch.

Surround yourself with the aromatic delights of fragrance.

Open your heart to the sensory experience of living.

Celebrate every day as it happens.   Live well.

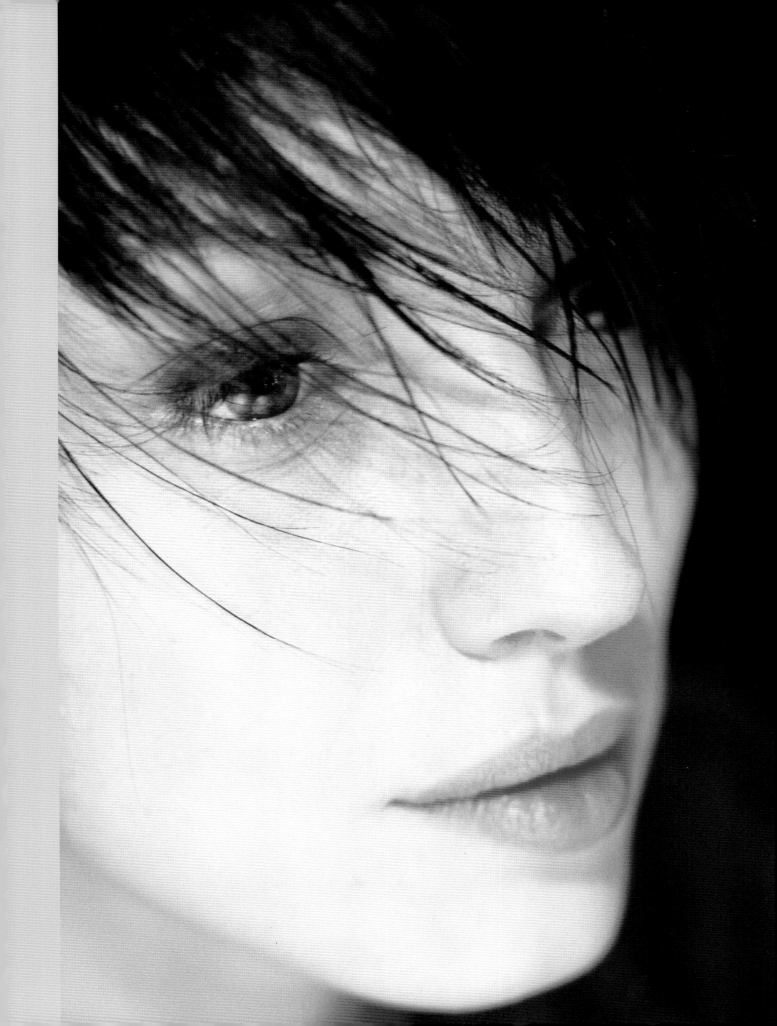

Carrier and essential oils recommended for use on the body

CHOOSE FROM THE FOLLOWING CARRIER OILS ALL OF WHICH CONTAIN BENEFITS, SUCH AS VITAMIN E AND IODINE

APRICOT KERNEL OIL is good for wrinkles and stretch marks and rich in vitamin A, which can increase the production of collagen.
COCONUT OIL acts as a cleanser and is good for oily skin.
GRAPESEED OIL is high in polyunsaturates and is particularly good for oily and combination skin types.
JOJOBA OIL regenerates all skin types and calms irritated skin.
MACADAMIA NUT OIL is very good for dry and ageing skin and is rich in vitamins A, E and F.
PEACH KERNEL OIL is nourishing and rich in vitamin A and is good for sun-damaged skin and stretchmarks.
SAFFLOWER OIL contains vitamins, minerals and proteins.
SOY BEAN OIL is good for oily skins. It contains polyunsaturates, acids, traces of chlorophyll and proteins.
SWEET ALMOND OIL is a clear pale yellow with a slight nutty note. It very good for softening dry, sensitive skin.
WHEATGERM OIL soothes, heals and smoothes the skin. It is an antioxidant, rich in vitamin E and phosphorous.

THE FOLLOWING OILS ARE A GOOD PLACE TO START YOUR ESSENTIAL OIL COLLECTION

As a general rule use a maximum of 8 drops essential oil to 10ml carrier oil for a facial or 12 drops to 30ml of carrier oil for a body massage. For baths add a maximum of 10 drops essential oil to 20ml carrier oil and in an oil burner add 4 drops to the water filled bowl.

BASIL is a nerve tonic that aids concentration and restores enthusiasm.
BERGAMOT is a sedative yet uplifting and helps allay anger and frustration. It should only be used in small amounts as it is a photosensitizer.
CHAMOMILE gently calms and soothes the nervous system, allaying fear and anxiety. It promotes relaxation and can help insomnia.
CARDAMOM is a restorative oil that alleviates fatigue and apathy.
CLARY SAGE is warming, relaxing, restoring and mind clearing. It is useful in cases of severe depression bringing lightness and peace whilst strengthening the nerves. It should be used with a grounding oil such as sandalwood, vetyver or juniper.
CYPRESS is a revitalising astringent and decongesting oil, that clears the head and aids concentration.
EUCALYPTUS is antiseptic and excellent for the respiratory system.
FRANKINCENSE is a very spiritual, calming, restorative oil ideal for meditation and best used with a grounding oil such as sandalwood, vetyver or juniper. It helps promote insight, peace and mental calm.
GERANIUM is relaxing, lifts the spirits and a superb hormonal rebalancer.
GINGER helps treat digestive disorders, travel sickness and strengthens the immune system.
GRAPEFRUIT has an uplifting reviving effect, relieving nervous tension. It is a cleansing, purifying oil that aids detoxification.
JASMINE is an aphrodisiac with a uniquely uplifting effect on emotions, calming the nerves and producing positive feelings of confidence. It has a soothing effect on muscular aches and tension and is great for alleviating labour pains.
JUNIPER stimulates the circulation and is a great mental clarifier and quells negativity. It is a revitalising oil that is a powerful detoxifier and diuretic. It is also antiseptic, astringent and healing.
LAVANDIN is a hybrid of blue and aspic lavender and has a perfume similar to camphor. It can provide a refreshing note for a tired mind.
LAVENDER is the universal panacea, it calms and soothes the body and soul. It is an antiseptic with unbelievable healing powers and is extremely effective in treating insomnia.
LEMON purifies and detoxifies the blood, helps lower blood pressure, stimulates the brain and helps you focus. It is refreshing and cooling helping clarify thought.
LEMONGRASS is a stimulating and powerful tonic with antibacterial properties. It is a very effective natural insect repellent.
LIME is uplifting, reviving, refreshing and can help relieve anxiety and fatigue. It stimulates the circulation to aid detoxification.
MANDARIN gives a sensation of serenity.
MARJORAM is warming, comfortingand sedative. It soothes the digestion and eases chest and respiratory problems.
MYRTLE detoxifies the tissues and acts as a decongestant.
NEROLI soothes calms and allays fear. It is good for insomnia and helps calm hyperactive children. Instills a feeling of peace.
NIAOULI is a very stimulating oil with healing and regenerating qualities. It is a powerful antiseptic.
PATCHOULI is an antidepressant, it helps to ground someone who is stressed and reduces the tendency to overthink. It is also an aphrodisiac.
PEPPERMINT is an energising and powerful decongestant, calms nausea and helps clear mental fog.
PETITGRAIN is an anti-depressent and makes a refreshing bath oil soothing sensitive skin.
PINE brings mental clarity as well as easing aches and pains and alleviating respiratory problems.

ROSE is a relaxing balancer of emotional disorders. It promotes inner poise and acts as a gentle opener for repressed emotions.

ROSEMARY stimulates slow circulation and is great for muscular aches. It stimulates the memory and enlivens the mind aiding concentration.

SANDALWOOD is a very relaxing sedative oil. It is calming, balancing and grounding. It helps you cope with stressful situations and is an aphrodisiac.

TEA TREE is an extremely versatile invigorating anti-bacterial oil that is also good in treating viral infections. It helps develop a positive mental outlook and can build confidence.

VETYVER, the oil of tranquillity, is deeply relaxing and beneficial for stress, anxiety and insomnia. It helps you cope in times of grief.

YLANG YLANG regulates adrenaline flow and relaxes the nervous system promoting a deep sense of wellbeing.

CAUTION

TWENTY-FOUR HOURS before using essential oils always conduct a patch test by using a little on the side of your face to make sure that no rash or soreness develops. Consult a trained aromatherapist if you are pregnant or taking medication.

NEVER APPLY essential oil directly to the skin (the only exception to this being lavender).

ESSENTIAL OILS, CANDLES AND VAPOURISERS should be kept out of reach of children and pets.

AVOID SKIN CONTACT with essential oils during pregnancy.

ESSENTIAL OILS should be stored in a dark, dry place.

DO NOT DRIVE after using frankincense or clary sage essential oils.

Skincare ingredients and terms

ALPHA HYDROXY ACIDS or AHAs speed up exfoliation by dissolving the glue that bonds dead skin cells to its surface, improving the colour and texture of the skin, unclogging pores and decreasing the build-up of blackheads. Long-term use prevents irritation and increases the skin's moisture-retaining abilities. The effects are fast, but benefits subside as soon as you stop use. Treat with caution and discontinue use at any sign of irritation; derived from natural ingredients such as grapes, apples, olives and milk, they can prove too harsh for sensitive skins. Wearing sunscreen when using AHAs is vital as the shedding of the top layer leaves the skin more exposed to sunlight.

ALPHA-LIPOIC ACID is a powerful naturally occurring anti-oxidant and anti-inflammatory that can increase a cell's metabolism boosting its capacity to heal. It is highly effective at reducing under eye puffiness.

ANTIOXIDANTS are vitamins and chemicals that combat damage from free radicals attacking the skin's collagen, cell membranes and lipid layer. Includes vitamins betacarotene, C and E and is found in plants.

BETA HYDROXY ACIDS are natural acids such as salicylic acid that work in a similar way to AHAs but they are less irritating. They are commonly used to treat acne, blackheads and blemishes and are used in spot treatments and toners. Use of sunscreen is a must and again they should be used with caution, as they are known irritants.

CERAMIDES are lipids found between skin cells that retain moisture and help stabilise the structure of the skin. They are deficient in dry skin.

CO-ENZYME Q-10 is considered essential for the body's cells, tissues and organs. It is oil-soluble and an excellent antioxidant. It is a popular alternative to retinoids and vitamin C as it is less irritating, however the results are also less apparent.

COLLAGEN/ELASTIN is required for skin elasticity and smoothness.

Over time their production slows down. As an ingredient, collagen attracts moisture and absorbs up to 30 times its weight in water.

ENZYMES are gentle non-irritating natural exfoliants and are derived from ingredients such as papaya.

HUMECTANTS attract moisture from the air to the surface of the skin and include glycerine, sorbitol, squalene and urea.

KINETIN contains a naturally occurring plant growth factor that keeps plant cells moist and healthy and retards their ageing. It reduces the appearance of fine lines, wrinkles and hyper-pigmentation, moisture loss and improves skin texture. It is a popular antioxidant.

LIPOSOMES deliver their moisturising cargo deep into the skin.

NATURAL MOISTURISING FACTORS or NMFs are naturally present in the skin and include sodium PCA, hyaluronic acid and linolenic acid.

PANTHENOL or pro-vitamin B5 can have a temporary skin plumping effect and is highly conditioning.

RETINOIDS (vitamin A derivatives) have a truly amazing effect on the skin, speeding up cell activity and unclogging pores. Vitamin A improves the skin's structure and increases collagen production. Tretinoins must be prescribed by a dermatologist and take up to 6 months to work. Retinol cream is weaker and available without prescription, it also reduces fine lines and skin discoloration but to a lesser extent. A stinging sensation is usually experienced upon application and skin may appear dry or flaky for the first few weeks of use. Skin may become photosensitive so they are best used at night and a sunscreen is necessary during the day.

VITAMIN C (L-ascorbic acid) has powerful antioxidants, it stimulates collagen production and aids healing. It is best worn under a sunscreen to boost the skin's resistance to UV damage. Irritation and stinging on application are known side effects.

SPACE.NK.apothecary

www.spacenk.com

LONDON

BROMPTON CROSS
307 Brompton Road, London SW3
tel: +44 (0)20 7589 8250

CANARY WHARF
Cabots Place West, London E14
tel: +44 (0)20 7719 1902

CHELSEA
307 Kings Road, London SW3
tel: +44 (0)20 7351 7209

CHISWICK
172 Chiswick High Road, London W4
tel: +44 (0)20 8994 3184

CITY
7 Bishopsgate Arcade, 185
Bishopsgate, London EC2
tel: +44 (0)20 7256 2303
145–147 Cheapside, London EC2
tel: +44 (0)20 7726 2060

COVENT GARDEN
4 Thomas Neals, 37 Earlham Street,
London WC2
tel: +44 (0)20 7379 7030

KENSINGTON
3 Kensington Church Street,
London W8
tel: +44 (0)20 7376 2870

KNIGHTSBRIDGE
SPACE.NK.apothecary@Harvey
Nichols, Knightsbridge, London SW1
tel: +44 (0)20 7201 8636

MARYLEBONE
83a Marylebone High Street,
London W1
tel: +44 (0)20 7486 8791

MAYFAIR
45–47 Brook Street, London W1
tel: +44 (0)20 7355 1727

NOTTING HILL
127–131 Westbourne Grove,
London W2
tel: +44 (0)20 7727 8063

ST. JOHNS WOOD
73 St. Johns Wood High Street,
London NW8
tel: +44 (0)20 7586 0607

BATH
10 New Bond Street, Bath BA1
tel: +44 (0)1225 482804

BELFAST
717 Lisburn Road, Belfast BT9
tel: +44 (0)28 90 663338

BIRMINGHAM
SPACE.NK.apothecary@Harvey
Nichols, The Mailbox, Birmingham B1
tel: +44 (0)121 616 6020

BLUEWATER
Lower Guild Hall, Bluewater,
Kent DA9
tel: +44 (0)1322 624562

EDINBURGH
97–103 George Street,
Edinburgh EH2
tel: +44 (0)131 225 6371

GLASGOW
36–37 Princes Square,
48 Buchanan Street, Glasgow G1
tel: +44 (0)141 248 7931

GUILDFORD
126 High Street, Guildford GU1
tel: +44 (0)1483 532654

LEEDS
63 Vicar Lane, Leeds LS1
tel: +44 (0)113 242 6606

MANCHESTER
102 The Dome, The Trafford Centre,
Manchester M17
tel: +44 (0)161 746 8669

Unit 15, Manchester Triangle,
Hanging Ditch, Manchester M4
tel: +44 (0)161 832 6220

RICHMOND
34 Hill Street, Richmond, Surrey TW9
tel: +44 (0)20 8940 4332

SPAce.NK.day spa

127 Westbourne Grove, London W2
tel: +44 (0)20 7727 8002

SPACE.NK.apothecary mail order

tel: +44 (0)870 169 9999

acupuncture

BRITISH ACUPUNCTURE COUNCIL
63 Jeddo Road, London W12
tel: +44 (0)20 8735 0400
www.acupuncture.org.uk

alexander technique

ALEXANDER TECHINQUE
INTERNATIONAL
8 Peters Place, Edinburgh EH3
tel: +44 (0)7071 880253
www.ati-net.com

SOCIETY OF TEACHERS OF THE
ALEXANDER TECHNIQUE
129 Camden Mews, London NW1
tel: +44 (0)20 7284 3338
www.stat.org.uk

aromatherapy

AROMATHERAPY TRADE COUNCIL
PO Box 387, Ipswich, Suffolk IP2
tel: +44 (0)1473 603630
www.a-t-c.org.uk

AROMATHERAPY ORGANISATIONS
COUNCIL
PO Box 19834, London SE25
tel: +44 (0)20 8251 7912

aromatherapy essential oils

AROMATHERAPY ASSOCIATES
PO Box 14981, London SW6
tel: +44 (0)20 7371 9878
www.aromatherapyassociates.com

G. BALDWIN & CO.
173 Walworth Road, London SE17
tel: +44 (0)20 7703 5550
www.baldwins.co.uk

ayurveda

AYURVEDIC MEDICAL ASSOCIATION UK
7 Park Crescent, London W1
tel: +44 (0)20 7631 0156

bach flower therapy

BACH FLOWER CENTRE
Mount Vernon, Sotwell, Wallingford,
Oxfordshire OX10
tel: +44 (0)1491 834678
www.bachcentre.com

bodywork

BOWEN ASSOCIATION
122 High Street, Earlshilton,
Leicestershire LE9
tel: +44 (0)1455 841800

HELLERWORK
Suite 211, Coppergate House,
16 Brunel Street, London E1
tel: +44 (0)20 7721 7770

ROLF INSTITUTE UK
PO Box 14793, London SW1
tel: +44 (0)20 7834 1493
www.rolf.org

TUI NA
Bodyharmonics Centre, 54 Fleckers
Drive, Hatherley, Cheltenham GL51
tel: +44 (0)1242 582168

ZERO BALANCING
10 Victoria Grove, Bridport,
Dorset DT6

chinese herbal medicine

REGISTER OF CHINESE HERBAL
MEDICINE
PO Box 400, Wembley, Middlesex HA9
tel: +44 (0)7000 790332
www.rchm.co.uk

BRITISH KANPO ASSOCIATION
Kailash Centre of Oriental Healing,
7 Newcourt Street, London NW8
tel: +44 (0)20 7722 3939
www.orientalhealing.co.uk

chiropractic

BRITISH CHIROPRACTIC ASSOCIATION
Blagrave House, 17 Blagrave Street,
Reading, Berkshire RG1
tel: +44 (0)118 950 5950
www.chiropractic-uk.co.uk

climbing

BRITISH MOUNTAINEERING COUNCIL
177 Burton Road, Manchester M20
tel: +44 (0)870 010 4878
www.thebmc.co.uk

cranial osteopathy

CHRISTIAN CHEMIN
1 Oldbury Place, London W1
tel: +44 (0)20 7486 2875

feldenkrais

FELDENKRAIS GUILD UK
PO Box 370, London N10
tel: +44 (0)7000 785506
www.feldenkrais.co.uk

hair styling

NICKY CLARKE
130 Mount Street, London W1
tel: +44 (0)20 7491 4700
www.nickyclarke.co.uk

ERROL DOUGLAS
18 Motcomb Street, London SW1
tel: +44 (0)20 7235 0110
www.erroldouglas.com

LUKE HERSHESON AT DANIEL
HERSHESON
45 Conduit Street, London W1
tel: +44 (0)20 7434 1797
www.danielhersheson.co.uk

hair colouring

DANIEL GALVIN
42–44 George Street, London W1
tel: +44 (0)20 7486 8601
www.daniel-galvin.co.uk

JO HANSFORD
198 Mount Street, London W1
tel: +44 (0)20 7495 7774
www.johansford.com

JOHN FRIEDA
4 Aldford Street, London W1
tel: +44 (0)20 7491 0840
www.johnfrieda.com

REAL
8 Cale Street, Chelsea Green,
London SW3
tel: +44 (0)20 7589 0877
www.realhair.co.uk

homeopathy

BRITISH HOMEOPATHIC
ASSOCIATION
15 Clerkenwell Close, London EC1
tel: +44 (0)20 7566 7800
www.trusthomeopathy.org

SOCIETY OF HOMEOPATHS
2 Artizan Road, Northampton NN1
tel: +44 (0)1604 621400
www.homeopathy-soh.org

manual lymphatic drainage

MLD UK
PO Box 14491, Glenrothes, Fife KY6
tel: +44 (0)1592 840799
www.mlduk.org.uk

massage

BRITISH MASSAGE THERAPY
COUNCIL
17 Rymers Lane, Oxford OX4
tel: +44 (0)1865 774123
www.bmtc.co.uk

nutritional supplements

NUTRI-CENTRE
7 Park Crescent, London W1
tel: +44 (0)20 7436 5122
www.nutricentre.com

nutrition

JANE CLARKE CONSULTANCY
29–30 Frith Street, London W1
tel: +44 (0)20 7437 3767

pedicures

IRIS CHAPPLE
3 Spanish Place, London W1
tel: +44 (0)20 7486 6001

MARCELA'S
7 Holland Street, London W8
tel: +44 (0)20 7938 1555

pilates

PILATES FOUNDATION UK
PO Box 36052, London SW16
tel: +44 (0)7071 781859
www.pilatesfoundation.com

reflexology

BRITISH REFLEXOLOGY ASSOCIATION
Monks Orchard, Whitbourne WR6
tel: +44 (0)1886 821207
www.britreflex.co.uk

THE KEET CLINIC
15 King Street, London WC2
tel: +44 (0)20 7240 1438
www.clsr.clara.net

reiki

REIKI ASSOCIATION
Cornbrook Bridge House, Ludlow SY8
tel: +44 (0)1584 891197
www.reikiassociation.org.uk

resistance bands

DYNA-BAND
Crown World Marketing, Drum
Grange, Nightingales Lane, Chalfont
St. Giles, Buckinghamshire HP8
tel: +44 (0)1494 764802
www.dynaband.co.uk

shiatsu

SACRED TRUST
PO Box 603, Bath BA1
tel: +44 (0) 1225 852615
www.sacredtrust.org

SHIATSU SOCIETY UK
Eastlands Courts, St Peters Road,
Rugby CV21
tel: +44 (0)1777 555051
www.shiatsu.org

skincare

ANNE SÉMONIN
108 rue du Faubourg Saint-Honoré,
75008 Paris
tel: +33 1 42 66 24 22

EVE LOM
2 Spanish Place, London W1
tel: +44 (0)20 7935 9988
www.evelom.co.uk

NICHOLAS LOWE
Harcourt House, Cavendish Square,
London W1
tel: +44 (0)20 7499 3223

DR JEAN-LOUIS SEBAGH
25 Wimpole Street, London W1
tel: +44 (0)20 7637 0548

t'ai chi

T'AI CHI ASSOCIATION UK
25 Arrol House,
Rockingham Street, London SE1
tel: +44 (0)20 7407 4775
www.taichiuk.co.uk

trichology

PHILIP KINGSLEY TRICHOLOGY
54 Green Street, London W1
tel: +44 (0)20 7629 4004
www.philipkingsley.co.uk

yoga

BRITISH WHEEL OF YOGA
25 Jermyn Street, Sleaford,
Lincolnshire NG34
tel: +44 (0)1529 306851
www.bwy.org.uk

yoga classes

IYENGAR YOGA INSTITUTE
223a Randolph Avenue, London W9
tel: +44 (0)20 7624 3080
www.iyi.org.uk

THE LIFE CENTRE
15 Edge Street, London W8
tel: +44 (0)20 7221 4602
www.thelifecentre.org

SIVANANDA YOGA VEDANTA
CENTRE
51 Felsham Road, London SW15
tel: +44 (0)20 8780 0160
www.sivananda.org/london

TRIYOGA
6 Erskine Road, London NW3
tel: +44 (0)20 7483 3344
www.triyoga.co.uk

YOGA THERAPY CENTRE
Royal Homeopathic Hospital,
60 Great Ormond Street,
London WC1
tel: +44 (0)20 7419 7195
www.yogatherapy.org

destination and day spas

AUSTRALIA

CAPE RETREAT
PO Box 810, Byron Bay,
New South Wales 2481
tel: +61 2 6684 1363
www.bayweb.com.au/caperetreat

COURAN COVE RESORT SPA AND
TOTAL LIVING CENTRE
PO Box 224, Runaway Bay,
Queensland 4216
tel: +61 7 5597 9000
www.couran-cove.com.au

DAINTREE ECO-LODGE AND SPA
20 Daintree Road, Daintree,
Queensland 4873
tel: +61 7 4098 6100
www.daintree-ecolodge.com.au

KANGAROO ISLAND RETREAT
PO Box 130, Kingscote, Kangaroo
Island, South Australia 5223
tel: +61 8 8553 5374
www.kihealthretreat.com

OBSERVATORY HOTEL SPA
89–113 Kent Street, Sydney 2000
tel: +61 2 9256 2229
www.observatoryhotel.com.au

SANCTUARY HOLISTIC RETREAT
PO Box 270, Bangalow, NSW 2479
tel: +61 2 6687 1216
www.sanctuary.org.au

SHIZUKA RYOKAN
8 Lakeside Drive, Hepburn Springs,
Victoria 3461
tel: +61 3 5348 2030
www.shizuka.com.au

SOLAR SPRINGS HEALTH RETREAT
96 Osborn Avenue, Bundanoon,
New South Wales 2578
tel: +61 2 4883 6027
www.solar.com.au

CANADA

ECHO VALLEY RANCH RESORT
PO Box 16, Clinton, Jesmond,
British Columbia
tel: +1 250 459 2386
www.evranch.com

MOUNTAIN TREK HEALTH SPA
PO Box 1352, Ainsworth Hot Springs,
British Columbia V0G 1AO
tel: +1 250 229 5636
www.hiking.com

SOLACE SPA AT FAIRMONT BANFF
SPRING HOTEL
PO Box 960, Banff, Alberta T1L 1J4
tel: +1 403 762 2211
www.fairmont.com

CARIBBEAN

AVEDA SPA
Strawberry Hill, Kingston, Jamaica
tel: +1 876 944 8400
www.aveda.com

LA CASA DE VIDA NATURAL
Rio Grande, Puerto Rico
tel: +1 787 887 4359
www.lacasaspa.com

MAGO ESTATE HOTEL
PO Box 247, Soufriere, St. Lucia
tel: +1 758 459 7352
www.mago-hotel.com

SHAMBHALA AT PARROT CAY
PO Box 164, Providenciales, Turks
and Caicos Islands, British West Indies
tel: +1 649 946 7788
www.parrot-cay.com

CYPRUS

THALASSA SPA AT ANASSA HOTEL
PO Box 66006, Polis CY-8830
tel: +357 6 888 000
www.thanoshotels.com

CZECH REPUBLIC

MARIENBAD AT HOTEL VILLA
BUTTERFLY
Hlavní trida 655, CZ-353 01
Mariánské Lázne
tel: +420 165 65 41 11
www.marienbad.cz

FRANCE

ANNE SÉMONIN SPA AT HÔTEL
LE BRISTOL
112 rue du Faubourg Saint Honoré,
75008 Paris
tel: +33 1 53 43 43 00
www.hotel-bristol.com

CAUDALIE INSTITUTE DE
VINOTHÉRAPIE AT LES SOURCES
DE CAUDALIE
Chemin de Smith Haut-Lafitte,
33650 Bordeaux-Martillac
tel: +33 5 57 83 83 83
www.sources-cadalie.com

DOMAINE DU ROYAL CLUB EVIAN
AT ROYAL PARC EVIAN
Rive Suid de Lac de Genève, 74500
Evian-Les-Bains
tel: +33 4 50 26 85 00
www.royalparcevian.com

INSTITUTE OF THALASSOTHERAPY
LOUISON BOBET AT HOTEL
MIRAMAR
13 rue Louison Bobet, 64200 Biarritz
tel: +33 5 59 41 30 01
www.sofitel.com

LANCÔME INSTITUT
29 rue du Fauborg Saint-Honoré,
75008 Paris
tel: +33 1 42 65 30 74
www.lancome.com

LES FERMES DE MARIE
Chemin de Riante Colline,
74120 Megève
tel: +33 4 50 93 03 10
www.fermesdemarie.com

LES THERMES MARINS DE
SAINT MALO
Grand plage du Sillon, BP 32,
35401 Saint Malo, Brittany
tel: +33 2 99 40 75 75
www.thalassosaintmalo.com

THALASSA QUIBERON
2 hôtels Sofitel et Ibis, Pointe de
Goulvars, BP 10802, 56170
Quiberon
tel: +33 2 97 50 20 00
www.thalassa.com

GERMANY

BRENNER'S PARK-HOTEL AND SPA
Schillerstraße 4–6,
76530 Baden Baden
tel: +49 72 21 90 00
www.brenners-park.de

INDIA

ANANDA SPA AT ANANDA IN THE
HIMALAYAS
Palace Estate, Narendra Nagar, Tehri,
Garhwal, Uttaranchal, Uttar Pradesh
tel: +91 137 82 7500
www.anandaspa.com

DHARMA AYURVEDIC HAVEN AT
KUMARAKOM LAKE RESORT
Kumarakom North PO, Pallichira,
Kottayam 686 566, Kerala
tel: +91 481 52 4900
www.klresort.com

INDUS VALLEY AYURVEDIC
CENTRE
Lalithadripura, Mysore PO Box 3,
Ittigegud, Mysore 570 010,
Karnataka
tel: +91 821 47 3437
www.ayurindus.com

JAI MAHAL PALACE
Jacob Road, Civil Lines, Jaipur 302
006, Rajasthan
tel: +91 141 22 3636
www.tajhotels.com

KAIRALI AYURVEDIC HEALTH RESORT
Kodumbu, Palakkad District
678551, Kerala
tel: +91 492 322 553
www.kairali.com

SPA AT RAJVILÂS
Goner Road, Jaipur 303 102,
Rajasthan
tel: +91 141 68 0101
www.oberoihotels.com

TAJ AYURVEDIC CENTRE AT
TAJ RESIDENCY HOTEL
PT Usha Road, Calicut 673 002, Kerala
tel: +91 495 76 5354
www.tajhotels.com

INDONESIA

BANYAN TREE BINTAN
Lagoi, Tanjong Said, Bintan Island
tel: +62 770 693 100
www.banyantree.com

JAMU TRADITIONAL SPA AT ALUM
KUL KUL RESORT
Jalan Pantai Kuta, Legian, Bali
tel: +62 361 763 701

JIMBARAN SPA AT FOUR SEASONS
RESORT BALI AT JIMBARAN BAY
Jimbaran, Denpasar 80361, Bali
tel: +62 361 701 010
www.fourseasons.com

MANDARA SPA AT THE CHEDI
Desa Melinggih Kelod, Payangan,
Gianyar 80572, Bali
tel: +62 361 975 963
www.mandaraspa-asia.com

MANDARA SPA AT THE IBAH
Campuhan, Ubud, Bali
tel: +62 361 974 466
www.mandaraspa-asia.com

OBEROI HOTEL, LOMBOK
Medana Beach, PO Box 1096,
Tanjung, Mataram 83001, West
Lombok, NTB, Malaysia
tel: +62 370 638 444
www.oberoihotels.com

SOURCE AT BEGAWAN GIRI ESTATE
PO Box 54, Ubud 80571, Bali
tel: +62 361 978 888
www.begawan.com

ISRAEL

CARMEL FOREST SPA RESORT
PO Box 9000, Haifa 31900
tel: +972 4 830 7888
www.isrotel.co.il

DEAD SEA SPA AT RADISSON
MORIAH PLAZA HOTEL
Dead Sea 86910
tel: +972 7 659 1591
www.radisson-moriah.co.il

ITALY

BAGNI SAN FILIPPO AT TERME
SAN FILIPPO HOTEL
53020 Bagni San Filippo (Siena),
Tuscany
tel: +39 0577 872 982
www.termesanfilippo.it

GRAND HOTEL TERME DI PETRIOLO
58040 Pari (Grosselo), Tuscany
tel: +39 0564 908 871

HOTEL DE RUSSIE
Via del Babuino 9, 00187 Rome
tel: +39 06 32 8881
www.hotelderussie.it

HOTEL TERME DI SATURNIA
58050 Saturnia (Grosselo), Tuscany
tel: +39 0564 600 800
www.termedisaturnia.it

MASSERIA SAN DOMENICO
72010 Savelletri di Fasano
(Brindisi), Puglia
tel: +39 080 482 79 90
www.imasseria.com

SATURNIA SPA AT PALAZZO ARZAGA
25080 Carzago di Calvagese della
Riviera, Brescia
tel: +39 030 680 600
www.palazzoarzaga.com

SPECCHIO DI VENERE AT MONASTERO
Pantelleria
tel: +39 02 581 861
www.monasteropantelleria.com

YOGAITALY
Villa Stampa, Lisciano Niccone,
Perugia
tel: +44 (0)20 7607 8885
www.yogaitaly.com

MALAYSIA

MANDARA SPA AT THE DATAI
Jalan Telek Datai, Palau Langkawi,
Kedah Darul Aman, Langkawi
tel: +60 4 959 2500
www.mandaraspa-asia.com

MEXICO

PUNTA SERENA
Km. 20 Carretera Federal 200,
Tenancatita, Municipio de la Huerta,
48989 Jalisco
tel: +52 335 15020/15100

RANCHO LA PUERTA
Tecate, Baja California
tel: +1 760 744 4222
www.rancholapuerta.com

SPA AT LAS VENTANAS AL PARAÍSO
Km. 19.5 Carretera Transpeninsular,
San Jose del Cabo, Baja California
sur 23400
tel: +52 624 144 0300
www.lasventanas.com

MOROCCO

AMANJENA HOTEL
Route de Ouarzazate, Marrakech
tel: +212 44 403 353
www.amanjena.com

SOUTH AFRICA

EARTH LODGE
Sabi Sabi, Kruger Park
tel: +27 11 483 3939
www.sabisabi.com

SÉRÉNITÉ WELLNESS CENTRE
PO Box 30097, Tokai, 7966 Cape Town
tel: +27 21 713 1760
www.serenite.co.za

SPAIN

THALASSO SPA AT MARBELLA
CLUB HOTEL
Bulevar Príncipe Alfonso von
Hohenlohe, 29600 Marbella, Malaga
tel: +34 95 282 2211
www.uk.marbellaclub.com

TRASIERRA
Crta. El Pedroso, Cazalla de la Sierra,
Seville

tel: +34 95 488 4324
www.patanegra.net

WINDFIRE YOGA
Can Am, Ibiza
tel: +34 97 118 7996
www.windfireyoga.com

SWITZERLAND

THERME VALS AT HOTEL THERME
7132 Vals/GR
tel: +41 81 926 8080
www.therme-vals.ch

VICTORIA-JUNGFRAU GRAND
HOTEL AND SPA
Höheveg 41, CH-3800 Interlaken
tel: +41 33 828 28 28
www.victoria-jungfrau.ch

THAILAND

BANYAN TREE PHUKET
33 Moo 4 Srisoonthorn Road,
Cherngtalay, Amphur Talang, Phuket
tel: +66 76 324 374
www.banyantree.com

ORIENTAL SPA AT THE MANDARIN
ORIENTAL BANGKOK
48 Oriental Avenue, Bangkok 10500
tel: +66 2 659 9000/439 7613
www.mandarin-oriental.com

SPA AT CHIVA-SOM
73/4 Petchkasem Road,
Hua Hin, Prachuab Khirikham 77110
tel: +66 32 536 536
www.chivasom.net

TURKEY

HUZUR VADISI
Gokceovacik, Gocek 48310, Fethiye
tel: +90 252 644 0008
www.huzurvadisi.com

UNITED KINGDOM

AGUA AT SANDERSON
50 Berners Street, London W1P 3AD
tel: +44 (0)20 7300 1414

BATH HOUSE AT ROYAL
CRESCENT HOTEL
16 Royal Crescent, Bath BA1 2LS
tel: +44 (0)1225 823333
www.royalcrescent.co.uk

BERKELEY HEALTH CLUB AND SPA
AT THE BERKELEY
Wilton Place, London SW1
tel: +44 (0)20 7201 1699
www.savoy-group.co.uk

BLISS SPA LONDON
60 Sloane Avenue, London SW3
tel: +44 (0)20 7584 3888
www.blissworld.com

CHAMPNEYS AT TRING
Wiggington Tring,
Hertfordshire HP23 6HY
tel: +44 (0)1441 863351
www.champneys.com

ELEMIS DAY SPA
2–3 Lancashire Court, London W1
tel: +44 (0)20 8909 5060
www.elemis.com

FOREST MERE HEALTH FARM
Liphook, Hampshire GU30 7JQ
tel: +44 (0)1428 726000
www.forestmere.co.uk

GRAYSHOTT HALL
Headley Road, Grayshott, Surrey
GU26 6JJ
tel: +44 (0)1428 602000
www.grayshott-hall.co.uk

HOAR CROSS HALL
Hoar Cross, Nr. Yoxall,
Staffordshire DE13
tel: +44 (0)1283 575671
www.hoarcross.uk
www.europeanayurveda.co.uk

LUCKNAM PARK
Colerne, Nr. Bath, Wiltshire SN14 8AZ
tel: +44 (0)1225 742777
www.lucknampark.co.uk

RAGDALE HALL HEALTH HYDRO
Ragdale Village, Nr. Melton Mowbray,
Leicestershire LE14 3PB
tel: +44 (0)1664 434831
www.ragdalehall.co.uk

SPA AT INCHYDONEY ISLAND
Clonakilty, West Cork, Ireland
tel: +353 23 33143
www.inchydoneyisland.com

SPA AT THE LYGON ARMS
Broadway, Worcestershire WR12 7DU

tel: +44 (0)1386 852255
www.the-lygon-arms.com

SPA AT MANDARIN ORIENTAL
66 Knightsbridge, London SW1
tel: +44 (0)20 7838 9888
www.mandarinoriental.com

USA

AGUA AT DELANO
1685 Collins Avenue, Miami Beach,
Florida FL 33139
tel: +1 305 672 2000

THE ASHRAM
2025 North McKain Street,
Calabasas, California 91372
tel: +1 818 222 6900
www.theashram.com

BEVERLY HOT SPRINGS
308 North Oxford Avenue,
Los Angeles, California 90004
tel: +1 323 724 7000
www.beverlyhotsprings.com

BLISS SPA 57
19 East 57th Street, 3rd floor,
NYC 10022, New York
tel: +1 212 219 8970
www.blissworld.com

BLISS SPA SOHO
568 Broadway, 2nd floor,
NYC 10012, New York
tel: +1 212 219 8970
www.blissworld.com

CAL-A-VIE SPA
29402 Spa Havens Way Vista, San
Diego, California 92084
tel: +1 760 945 2055
www.cal-a-vie.com

CANYON RANCH
Tucson, Arizona
tel: +1 800 742 9000
www.canyonranch.com

CARAPAN URBAN SPA AND STORE
5 West 16th Street, Garden level,
NY 10011, New York
tel: +1 212 633 6220
www.carapan.com

DUNTON HOT SPRINGS
PO Box 818, Dolores, Colorado 81323

tel: +1 970 882 4800
www.duntonhotsprings.com

ESALEN INSTITUTE
Highway 1, Big Sur, California
93920-9616
tel: +1 831 667 3000
www.esalen.org

GOLDEN DOOR
PO Box 463077, Escondido,
California 92046-3077
tel: +1 760 744 5007
www.goldendoor.com

THE LODGE AT SKYLONDA
16350 Skyline Boulevard, Woodside,
California 94062
tel: +1 650 851 6625
www.skylondalodge.com

MII AMO SPA
525 Boynton Canyon Road, Sedona,
Arizona 86336
tel: +1 888 749 2137
www.miiamo.com

MIRAVAL RESORT AND SPA
Tucson, Arizona
tel: +1 800 232 3969
www.miravalresort.com

OJAI VALLEY INN AND SPA
Country Club Road, Ojai, California
93023
tel: +1 805 646 1111
www.ojairesort.com

POST RANCH INN
Highway 1, PO Box 219, Big Sur,
California 93920
tel: +1 831 667 2200
www.postranchinn.com

SOHO SANCTUARY
119 Mercer Street, 3rd Floor, NY
10012, New York
tel: +1 212 334 5550
www.sohosanctuary.com

SPA MYSTIQUE AT THE CENTURY
PLAZA HOTEL
2025 Avenue of the Star, Century
City, Los Angeles, California 90067-
4696
tel: +1 310 551 3251
www.spamystique.com

TEN THOUSAND WAVES
PO Box 10200, Sante Fe, New
Mexico 87504
tel: +1 505 992 5025
www.tenthousandwaves.com

TWO BUNCH PALMS AT NATURAL
HOT SPRINGS RESORT AND SPA
67–425 Two Bunch Palms Trail,
Desert Hot Springs, California 92240
tel: +1 760 329 8791
www.twobunchpalms.com

recommended reading

Aroma: The Cultural History of Smell,
Constance Classen, David Honer and
Anthony Synott (Routledge)
Ayurveda: The Science of Self-healing,
Dr V. Lad (Motilal Banarsidass)
Bobbi Brown Beauty, Bobbi Brown
and AnneMarie Iverson (Ebury Press)
The Book of the Bath, François de
Bonneville (Thames and Hudson)
Chi Kung, Eleanor McKenzie (Hamlyn)
Colours of the Soul, June MacLeod
(Piatkus Books)
Colour Therapy, Pauline Wills (Element)
Essence and Alchemy, Mandy Aftel
(Bloomsbury)
The Healthy Home, Gina Lazenby
(Conran Octopus)
The Integrated Health Bible, Dr
Mosaraf Ali (Vermilion)
Juice Fasting and Detoxification,
Steve Meyerowitz (Book Publishing Co)
Living Zen, Michael Paul (Frances Lincoln)
Meditation for Life, Martine
Batchelor (Frances Lincoln)
The Okinawa Program, Bradley J.
Willcox, D. Craig Willcox and Makoto
Suzuki (Three Rivers Press)
Perfume, Susan Irvine (Aurum Press)
Sacred Spaces, Denise Linn (Rider)
Sensual Home, Ilse Crawford (Quadrille)
Superjuice, Michael van Straten
(Mitchell Beazley)
Thinking Body, Dancing Mind,
Chungliang Al Huang and Jerry
Lynch (Bantam Books)
Yoga: A Gem for Women, Geeta S.
Iyengar (Timeless Books)
Yoga and Ayurveda, David Frawley
(Lotus Light)

index

abhyanga massage 127
acupuncture 126
air-conditioned offices 43
air travel 139
alcohol consumption 43, 98
Alexander technique 120
antioxidants 24, 28, 29, 43, 153
aqua therapies 120
aromatherapy massage 124, 144, 147
  see also oils, essential
ashtanga yoga 13
astringents 44, 45
Ayurvedic therapies 127, 144

bad breath 57
basil/basil oil 30, 44, 57, 152
bathing 18, 75, 85, 96-97
  in essential oils 21, 70, 76, 97,
    98, 14
  in milk 47
bathrooms 96, 113, 150
bedrooms 113
bergamot oil 13, 14, 69, 152
blackheads, removing 44
blusher, applying 53, 57
body brushing, dry 17
body scrubs 18, 47
brahmari 119
breakfasts 13
breath control exercises 119–20
breath-counting meditation 90
breathing, deep 38, 116
broccoli 29, 30
brushes, make-up 57

cabbage 29
callisthenics 25
candle meditation 93
candlelight 66, 97
candles, scented 66, 69
carbohydrates 27
carrots/carrot juice 30, 31
chamomile/chamomile oil 65, 97,
  152
chamomile tea 38
chi gong 120
cholesterol 24, 27, 29
cinnamon 27, 30
citrus fruits/oils 13, 14, 20, 28, 29

clary sage oil 14, 152
cleansers, skin 44
coconut oil 58
colours: and mood 8, 35, 66, 86
concealer, applying 53
concentration, boosting 14
conditioners, hair 60
craniosacral therapy 127

dandruff 60
Dead Sea salts 18, 21, 144
dental care 57
deodorants 14
detox diet 128, 130–31
diet 8, 26, 27, 38, 58
  yogic 128, 130–31
digestive aids 27, 38, 57

energy boosting 13, 17, 18, 20–21
  and exercise 24–25
  and food 26–30, 31
eucalyptus oil 14, 65, 152
exercise 13, 17, 24–25, 43, 98,
  116, 136, 149
exfoliation 17, 20, 45, 147
eyes 54
  applying eyeliner 54–55, 57, 79
  applying mascara 55, 79
  applying shadow 55, 57, 79
  curling eyelashes 55, 79
  puffiness 54
  shaping eyebrows 54

face masks 45
face powder, using 53
facial scrubs 45
facials 45
fasting 131
fats 27
feet, caring for 50
fennel 27, 57
fibre, dietary 27, 29
fingernails, care of 48
fish 27
flavonoids 28, 29
flaxseed 27, 29
flexibility, increasing 25
flower remedies 127
food see diet
footcare 50
foundation, applying 53, 79
free radicals 29, 43
fruit/fruit juices 28, 29, 30, 35, 131

gardens 107, 150
garlic 29
geranium oil 38, 152
ginger 27, 30, 152
grapes 29

hair and haircare 58, 139, 149
  changing colour 61
  changing style 60
  drying 61
  rinses 60
  styling products 61
  washing and conditioning 60
hallways 113
hands, care of 48
health programmes 144
herbal teas and tisanes 27, 38,
  101, 131
holidays 135, 136, 139, 140
holistic health training 143
home environments 35, 36, 66, 85,
  86, 108, 110, 112, 113
homeopathy 127
hormone replacement therapy 43
hydrotherapy 144

incense burning 69
Indian head massage 127

jasmine oil 26, 44, 65, 69, 152
jin shin jyutsu 126
juices, fruit and vegetable 30, 31, 131

kapalabhati 119
kewra oil 69
khus 69
kinesiology 127
kitchens 113

la stone therapy 124
laughter 8, 13
lavender/lavender oil 38, 85, 97, 152
legumes 29
lemongrass oil 26, 152
lemons/lemon oil 14, 28, 29, 152
lime oil 13, 14, 38, 152
lips 56
  applying lipstick and lipliner 56,
    57, 79
  chapped 56
living rooms 113
lunches 38
lymphatic drainage massage 124

make-up, applying 53; see also
  eyes; lips
  for night-time 78–79
manicure, home 48
mantra meditation 93
marjoram/marjoram oil 14, 30, 97, 152
mascara, applying 55
massage 13, 20–21
  aromatherapy 124, 144, 147
  Ayurvedic 127
  deep tissue 124
  la stone therapy 124
  lymphatic drainage 124
  scalp 60
  sports 124
  Swedish 124
  Thai 126
  tui na 126
meditation 38, 86, 89, 90, 93, 116,
  143
memory boosting 14
minerals 27, 28
moisturisers 45
movement therapies 116
mud treatments 144
music 13, 35, 38, 66, 86, 97, 98, 108

nails, care of 48, 50, 79
naturopathy 127
neroli oil 69, 152

oatmeal body scrub 47
oestrogen 43
offices 14, 38, 43, 113
oils, essential 14, 35, 45, 65, 152–53
  appetite-suppressing 26
  for bathing 13, 21, 47, 70, 97, 98
  for massage 20–21
  vaporising 26, 69
oils, facial 45
omega-3 fat 27
onions 29
orange oil 26

panchakarma 127
patchouli oil 69, 152
pedicure, home 50
peppermint oil 26, 65, 152
peppermint tea 38
perfumes 72–73
Pilates 25, 120
plants 107
polarity therapy 127

powder, face 53
powder brushes 57
pranayama 119
protein 27

reflexology 126
reiki 127
relaxation 38, 116; *see also* meditation
retinoids 153
retreats 135, 140, 143
rosemary/rosemary oil 14, 27, 38, 65, 152
roses/rose oil 26, 38, 69, 97, 152
rosewater sprays 38
sandalwood oil 38, 153
scents 13, 14, 65, 69, 70, 72–73
serotonin 43
shampoos 60
shiatsu 126

shirodhara 127
showering 13, 18, 20
skin/skincare 42–45, 149, 153
    body scrubs 18, 47
    exfoliation 17, 20, 45, 147
    milk bath 47
sleep 85, 98, 101
sodium laurel sulfate 20
sounds 97; *see also* music
soy beans/soy products 29
spas 135, 140, 144, 147
spinach 30
sports 136; *see also* exercise
spots 43
stress 43, 57, 112
    reducing 24, 38, 89, 116, 135
sugars 26–27
sun, protection against 43, 139
t'ai chi 120
tangerine oil 26, 38

tea tree oil 14, 153
teas, herbal 27, 38, 131
teeth, caring for 57
Thai massage 126
thalassotherapy centres 144
threading (facial hair removal) 54
tisanes *see* herbal teas and tisanes
toenails, care of 50
tomatoes: for skincare 44
toners 45
toothpastes 57
touch 97, 110
trataka 93
travel sickness, preventing 139
tui na 126
turmeric 98

ujjayi breathing 119

vanilla oil 26, 65

vegetables/vegetable juices 28, 29, 30, 31, 35, 131
visualisation 116
vitamins 27, 28, 30, 43, 58, 131, 153

water, importance of 27, 35, 43, 130–31
watercress 30
weight-management programmes 144
weight training 24–25
wrinkles 43, 44

yeast, brewer's 58
ylang ylang oil 69, 153
yoga 13, 25, 38, 120–21, 122–23
yogic diet 128, 130–31

Zen 106–107

author's acknowledgments

Thank you to Alison Cathie who finally persuaded me to put pen to paper in what became a personal quest for self-discovery and improvement, Jane O'Shea who provided necessary and invaluable focus, Lisa Pendreigh for her endless hard work and Mary Evans for art directing the vision. A big thank you to Nadine Bazar, your patience is limitless.

This work would not have been possible without the invaluable knowledge and advice gleaned from the experts I have had the good fortune to meet in all walks of life over the years – thank you for sharing with me.

And finally a big thank you to family and friends for being there unconditionally.

This book is dedicated to Peter, you opened my eyes and changed my thinking. Thank you.

picture credits

2 Rex Features; 4 left *Marie France*/Dolores Marat; 4 centre Photonica/Jen Haas; 4 right Sølve Sundsbø; 5 far left Tessa Traeger; 5 left Photonica/Mia Klein; 5 centre Tessa Traeger; 5 right The Interior Archive/Eric Morin; 5 far right Bohnchang Koo; 6 *Marie France*/Dolores Marat; 12 Photonica/Jen Haas; 14–15 Camera Press/*Sarie Visi*; 16 Luca Tettoni Photography; 19 Red Cover/*Maisons Coté Sud*/Frederic Vasseur; 22–23 Photonica/Yukari Ochiai; 25 Gettyimages/Chris Cole; 27 *Deco Idées*/Gino Campens/stylist Kat de Baerdemaeker; 28 Sue Snell; 31 The Condé Nast Publications/*Vogue Entertaining Cookbook*/William Meppem; 34 Sølve Sundsbø; 36–37 *Maison Madame Figaro*/Bernard Langenstein; 39 Gettyimages/Anne-Marie Weber; 40–41 robertharding.com; 42 Sanoma Syndication/Arjaan Hamel; 46–47 Narratives/Polly Wreford; 49 Sølve Sundsbø; 51 IPC Syndication/© *Living Etc.*/David Clerihew; 52 Camera Press/Sarie Visi; 55 ImageState; 56 IPC Syndication/© *Essentials*/Annie Johnston; 59 *Marie Claire Maison*/François Deconinck; 61 Gettyimages/Vincent Besnault; 64 Tessa Traeger; 67 Camera Press/*Viva*; 68 Andrea Ferrari/interior designer Isabella Sodi; 71 Gettyimages/Deborah Jaffe; 74 Magnum/Ferdinando Scianna; 77 Red Cover/*Maisons Coté Sud*/Bernard Touillon; 78–79 The Interior Archive/James Wedge; 80-81 ImageState; 84 Photonica/Mia Klein; 87 Minh & Wass; 88 Narratives/Jan Baldwin; 91 Sanoma Syndication/Conny Hofmans; 92 Sølve Sundsbø; 94–95 Photonica/Shinichi Eguchi; 99 Red Cover/*Maisons Coté Sud*/Frederic Vasseur; 100 Minh & Wass; 104-105 Tessa Traeger; 106–107 Topham Picturepoint; 108–109 Bruno Helbling/architect Samuel Lerch/interior designer Benjamin Thut; 111 Guy Obijn; 112–113 Craig Fraser/architects Richard Tremeer & John Jacobson/interior design Cheryl Cowley; 114–115 Hutchison Library/Felix Greene; 117 Sanoma Syndication/Hotze Eisma; 118 Francine Fleischer/photograph courtesy of Parrot Cay Resort; 120 Impact Photos/Keith Cardwell; 123 The Condé Nast Publications Ltd/Robert Erdmann © *Vogue*; 125 ImageState; 126 The Condé Nast Publications Ltd/Anne Menke © *Condé Nast Traveller*; 129 *Marie Claire Maison*/Marc Montezin; 130 IPC Syndication/© *Country Homes & Interiors*/Sandra Lane; 134 The Interior Archive/Eric Morin; 137 Gettyimages/Brian Bailey; 138 Red Cover/*Maisons Coté Sud*/Bernard Touillon; 141 Gettyimages/Preston-Schlebusch; 142–143 Margherita Spiluttini/architect Peter Zumthor; 145 Powerstockzefa; 146 *Famili*/S Martinelli; 148 Bohnchang Koo; 151 Limelight/Jean Philippe Lacube.